LECTURE NOTES ON
OPHTHALMOLOGY

LECTURE NOTES ON
OPHTHALMOLOGY

Patrick D. Trevor-Roper
M.A., M.D., B.Chir. (Cantab)., F.R.C.S., D.O.M.S. (Eng.)
Consultant Ophthalmic Surgeon
Westminster Hospital and
Moorfields Eye Hospital

SIXTH EDITION

BLACKWELL
SCIENTIFIC PUBLICATIONS
OXFORD LONDON EDINBURGH
BOSTON MELBOURNE

To E. F. K.

First published 1960
Reprinted 1961, 1963
Second edition 1965
Third edition 1968
Fourth edition 1971
Fifth edition 1974
Reprinted 1976
Sixth edition 1980
Spanish edition 1978

Printed in Great Britain at
The Alden Press, Oxford
and bound by
Kemp Hall Bindery, Oxford

DISTRIBUTORS

USA
    Blackwell Mosby Book Distributors
    11830 Westline Industrial Drive
    St Louis, Missouri 63141

Canada
    Blackwell Mosby Book Distributors
    120 Melford Drive, Scarborough
    Ontario, M1B 2X4

Australia
    Blackwell Scientific Book
    Distributors
    214 Berkeley Street, Carlton
    Victoria 3053

British Library
Cataloguing in Publication Data

Trevor-Roper, Patrick Dacre
    Lecture notes on ophthalmolo-
gy.—6th ed.
    1. Eye—Diseases and defects
    I. Title
    617.7   RE46

ISBN 0-632-00642-0

CONTENTS

PREFACE TO SIXTH EDITION

This sixth edition introduces widespread amendments, which reflect the ever-changing face of ophthalmic practice. To keep abreast of changes in examination techniques, I have added an appendix of Multiple Choice Questions, as well as a short glossary, for both of which I am grateful to the help and patience of Dr Stuart Pinkerton, and which I hope will ease the passage of the hard-pressed student.

3 Park Square West,   Patrick Trevor-Roper
London NW1

PREFACE TO FIRST EDITION

This little guide does not presume to tell the medical student all that he needs to know about ophthalmology, for there are many larger books that do. But the medical curriculum becomes yearly more congested, while ophthalmology, still the 'Cinderella' of medicine, is generally left until the last, and only too readily goes by default. So it is to these harrassed final-year students that the book is principally offered, in the sincere hope that they will find it useful; for nearly all eye diseases are recognized quite simply by their appearance, and a guide to ophthalmology need be little more than a gallery of pictures, linked by lecture notes.

My second excuse for publishing these lecture notes is a desire I have always had to escape from the traditional textbook presentation of ophthalmology as a string of small isolated diseases, with long unfamiliar names, and a host of eponyms. To the nineteenth-century empiricist, it seemed proper to classify a long succession of ocular structures, all of which emerged as isolated brackets for yet another sub-catalogue of small and equally isolated diseases. Surely it is time now to try and harness these miscellaneous ailments not in terms of their diverse morphology, but in simpler clinical patterns; not as the microscopist lists them, but in the different ways that eye diseases present. For this, after all, is how the student will soon be meeting them.

I am well aware of the many inadequacies and omissions in this form of presentation, but if the belaboured student finds these lecture notes at least more readable, and therefore more memorable, than the prolix and time-honoured pattern, perhaps I will be justified.

ACKNOWLEDGEMENTS

My first thanks are due to my former teacher and colleague at Westminster Medical School, Mr E.F.King, who kindly checked the first edition of this book in proof. Other friends have given valued guidance over each of the subsequent versions.

For the illustrations, I am particularly indebted to Dr P. Hansell's Department of Medical Illustrations at the Institute of Ophthalmology, where most of the original drawings and photographs were prepared, many of these having already appeared in my textbook *The Eye and its Disorders*, also published by Blackwell Scientific Publications. For the loan of other blocks I am indebted to H. K. Lewis & Co Ltd (Wolff's *Anatomy of the Eye*, Figs. 2.1 and 8.3); Ballière, Tindall & Co Ltd (May and Worth's *Diseases of the Eye*, by T. K. Lyle and A. G. Cross, Fig. 6.1) Longmans, Green & Co Ltd (Gray's *Anatomy*, Fig. 2.12); H. Kimpton (*Textbook of Ophthalmology*, by Sir S. Duke-Elder, Fig. 8.4.

CHAPTER 1
INTRODUCTION

To the ancients the eye was the gateway for the soul, and to the physician of today that modest organ indeed serves as a window through which the evidence can be seen of half the maladies to which man is heir. But the diseases specific to the eye itself are no less important, for the eye is exposed and vulnerable, and because man is primarily a visually-motivated machine, with an especial dread of anything that might lead to blindness.

The investigation of eye diseases is happily quite a simple affair. In the main there are only two presenting symptoms—loss of sight and pain; and since the affected tissues are so readily inspected, the front by a magnifying lens, and the back by the ophthalmoscope, the patient's subjective interpretation of his symptoms is of minor importance, and the diagnosis thus based on the objective findings of the surgeon can be comfortably exact and secure.

Eye diseases are readily grouped into two very different categories, separated by the tough outer wall of the eyeball.

The *external* diseases—such as those of lids and conjunctiva—behave like the many familiar diseases of skin and mucosa elsewhere in the body; they invite direct inspection, and are easily approached for a culture or biopsy; and they are equally amenable to topical treatment, since the drugs can be placed directly onto the affected cells, with rarely any danger of systemic poisoning, with maximal economy and with maximal ease; while minor operations again have easy access, rarely become infected, heal readily, and the results are most rewarding.

It is a very different matter when we deal with the *internal* eye diseases—those which affect the structures within that fibrous envelope. They can less easily be inspected, perhaps only darkly through a semi-opaque cornea or lens. They can be reached only with difficulty and danger for biopsy or culture, and even then the histological changes are often inconclusive, and the cultures negative; with the result that the aetiology of most internal eye diseases remains quite obscure. And finally, they are inaccessible for treatment, since—even where an effective agent exists—the corneo-sclera forms an impenetrable barrier to nearly all topical applications that are foreign to the body.

*

Before considering the specific diseases of the eye, a few words are needed about the eye itself, and the form and function of its several parts.

The **eyeball**, a sphere nearly an inch in diameter, lies suspended within the fat which fills the orbit; it is protected by the four converging bony orbital walls, but unprotected anteriorly where the convex corneal window lies. The latter is screened by the upper and, to a small extent, the lower eyelids (Fig. 1.1); while a vestigial third eyelid lies immobile in the inner angle as a conjunctival fold (the 'plica semilunaris'), containing a fatty nodule known as the caruncle.

The **sclera** is the fibrous envelope of the eyeball. Its anterior aperture, 10 mm. in diameter, is occupied by the **cornea**, which differs in being transparent, avascular and slightly more convex than the Sclera. Since the cornea is exposed to all manner of traumata and of exogenous pathogens, its principal pathology lies in its liability to ulcerate; and even if such ulcers rarely penetrate the whole corneal thickness, they leave opaque scars which, if centrally placed, may seriously impair the sight.

The cornea consists of a thin epithelium (five cell layers, corresponding to the three inner cell strata of the epidermis), a thick stroma of laminated fibre-bundles which continue into the sclera with little histological change, and a single layer of endothelial cells in contact with the aqueous humour (Fig. 1.2).

Lining the inner surface of the sclera is a mesodermal sheet known as the **'uveal tract'**, (Fig 1.2), loaded with blood-vessels and containing at its anterior end the unstriated intra-ocular muscles. Posteriorly this thin sheet is known as the **choroid**, and between its lattice of vessels lies a variable amount of pigment, so that on ophthalmoscopy of dark-skinned races the fundus appears chocolate in colour (Plate 1, following p. 60); while in albinos the absence of pigment both exposes the wide interlacing choroidal vessels, and in the polygonal spaces between them reveals the white sclera (Plate 2, following p. 60).

The choroid reaches forward to within 6 mm of the corneo-scleral junction, and there the uveal tract becomes swollen by the fibres of the ciliary muscle, so that this intermediate zone is known as the **ciliary body** (Fig. 1.2 and 1.3). From ridges on the inner surface of the ciliary body, fine fibres converge to the rim of the lens as its suspensory ligament.

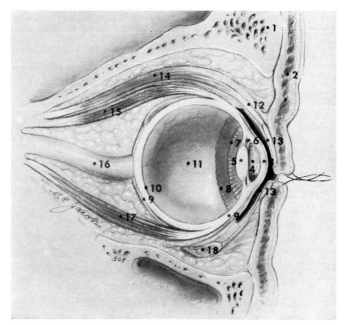

Fig. 1.1. Vertical section of eyeball within the orbit. (from *Medical Radiography and Photography*, Courtesy of Camille Hill Killan.)

1. Frontal bone (orbital rim).	11. Vitreous space.
2. Orbicularis oculi muscle.	12. Muller's muscle (involuntary;
3. Cornea.	connecting L.P.S. and upper
4. Anterior chamber.	tarsal plate).
5. Lens.	13. Tarsal conjunctiva.
6. Iris Root.	14. Levator palpebrae superioris
7. Ciliary body.	muscle.
8. Ora serrata (anterior edge of	15. Superior rectus muscle.
retina)	16. Optic nerve.
9. Sclera.	17. Inferior rectus muscle.
10. Choroid and retina.	18. Inferior oblique muscle.

From the anterior margin of the ciliary body, the uveal tract is continued as the **iris**, which, no longer clinging to the corneoscleral envelope, lies as a coronal sheet behind the cornea. Its muscles are disposed as a pupillary sphincter, encircling the pupillary rim, and a sheet of radiating fibres that forms the pupillary dilator. Before birth the pupil is occluded by vascular mesoderm, and even in later life fine strands of a 'persistent pupillary membrane' can often be seen. The complex developmental history of the eye yields a corresponding harvest of other congenital anomalies, and in the iris these readily provoke attention. Thus a sector-shaped gap or 'coloboma' is not uncommon, which may extend backwards to involve the ciliary body and choroid; or the iris may be totally absent ('aniridia'), or of a different colour from its fellow ('heterchromia'). In albinos the iris is translucent and pink, since its only remaining pigment is haemoglobin.

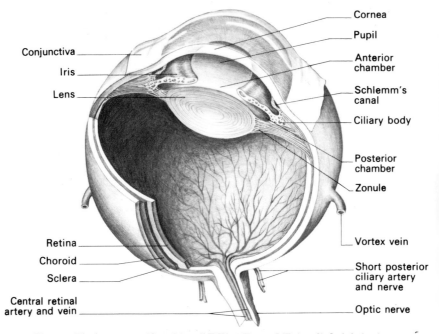

Fig. 1.2. The human eye (from Newell F.W. & Ernest J.T. (1978) *Ophthalmology: Principles and Concepts*, 4th edn. St Louis: C.V. Mosby Co).

The **aqueous humour**, whose physiology is very similar to that of the cerebrospinal fluid, oozes from the capillaries of the iris and ciliary muscle, and circulates from the 'posterior chamber' (lying behind the iris) to reach the recesses of the 'anterior chamber' (between iris and cornea), whence it disperses into the episcleral veins via an encircling 'canal of Schlemm'.

The **lens** consists of a clear viscous matrix within a thin elastic capsule; and it lies in contact with the posterior surface of the iris suspended by its 'ligament' from the ciliary body. The ciliary muscle acts primarily as sphincter, so that, on contraction, it relaxes the suspensory ligament, and

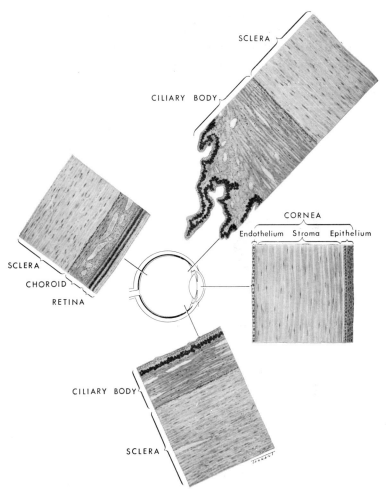

Fig. 1.3. Histology of the coats of the eyeball.

hence also the elastic lens capsule, with the result that the lens becomes more spherical, and thus focuses for near-vision.

Lining the inner surface of the choroid is the **retina**, with its rods and cones up against the choroidal surface, and the various cell relays running forwards and inwards, so that the fibres of the innermost 'ganglion cells' lie in contact with the vitreous surface. These fibres course (along with the retinal vessels) towards the optic nerve-head, or 'optic disc', and thence as the fibres of the optic nerve* back through the chiasma to their next relay in the lateral geniculate body. The fibres from the temporal half of the retina (carrying impulses from the nasal half of the visual field of that eye) come to lie laterally in the optic nerve, so that a lesion to the lateral side of the nerve will cause a loss of the nasal visual field. At the chiasma, the medial fibres cross over, and an interruption of the crossing fibres (as by a pituitary tumour) thus causes a bi-temporal hemianopia. Further back a lesion of the right optic tract, radiations or occipital cortex will cause a left homonymous hemianopia (loss of the left half-field of each eye); with the upper quadrant of the field principally impaired when the lower fibres of tract, radiations or cortex are principally damaged and vice-versa.

GENERAL EXAMINATION

The general examination of the eye demands little beyond a good light, a magnifying lens ('loupe'), and an ophthalmoscope; and the principles of examination are really self-evident. One should start by noting the 'setting' of the two eyes, any asymmetry of their position, size or colour, particularly any difference in size of the palpebral aperture (as from a relative ptosis, or proptosis) or in size of the pupil. Then should follow a check of the pupil reactions to light—direct and consensual (from illumination of the fellow-eye) and to accommodation-convergence; and a check of the eye-movements, by fixing the patient's head with one hand and asking him to watch one's finger as it travels upward, downward, to left and to right (the relative positions of the two bright corneal light-reflections will betray an eye that lags in any particular direction of gaze). Then one turns to the individual eyes, checking in turn each of the structures from before backwards (lids, conjunctiva, cornea, iris and pupil, lens, and then with the ophthalmoscope,† the fundus). Finally, the intra-

---

* These fibres have no medullary sheath until they reach the optic nerve-head. Occasionally medullation transgresses a little onto the retinal surface, as a striking but harmless congenital anomaly (Plate 7c, following p. 60).
† *Notes on basic Technique.* Use right eye for right eye of patient and vice-versa, placing left hand on patient's forehead, with thumb elevating upper lid. Patient fixes eyes on object straight ahead. Surgeon holds Ophthalmoscope (without any lens interposed) up against his nose (keeping his other eye open if possible), gradually approaching patient along a line about 15° lateral to his direction of fixation, so that the patient's optic disc should be brought immediately into view (and promptly assessed, lest it is never seen again!). If it is out of focus, rotate the wheel of the ophthalmoscope using increasingly strong concave lenses: if still out of focus, suspect lens or vitreous opacities. Then follow down the four vascular

ocular pressure can be roughly checked by fluctuating the down-turned eye between one's two fore-fingers and contrasting its impressibility with that of its fellow or a normal eye (Fig. 3.11).

Eversion of the upper lid over a finger or glass rod (Fig. 1.4) will allow inspection of the under surface of the upper lid. This is most easily done by standing behind the patient, who is told to look at the floor, and then by

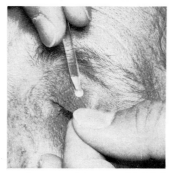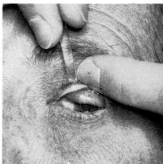

Fig. 1.4. Eversion of the upper lid. (Wybar.)

pulling the upper lashes forwards and upwards, so that the lid is rolled over the upper edge of its tarsal plate, which is meanwhile pressed backwards by the forefinger of the other hand. Foreign particles often become caught in the horizontal groove beneath the upper lid, and, when exposed in this way, can readily be removed.

Visual acuity

(Fig. 1.5) is the most important subjective examination, normally tested by using 'Snellen's types', at a distance of 6 metres (to exclude all but a negligible amount of accommodation). Vision is expressed as a fraction of the normal, the smallest letter usually visible without effort is thus '6/6'; if the patient can only see the letter twice its size, his visual acuity is '6/12'; while the largest letter usually displayed (10 times its size, which would thus be comfortably visible to the normal-sighted at 60 metres distance) designates a visual acuity of '6/60'. Still poorer vision is indicated by his

trunks looking for retinopathy; and finally check the macula (if elusive, ask the patient to look straight into the light). Inspection of the macula or fundus periphery is difficult unless the pupil has been dilated by mydriatic drops, such as tropicamide 0·5%.

capacity to count fingers ('C.F.'), see hand movements ('H.M.') and finally just to perceive light (P.L.'). Near vision is similarly tested by a card bearing graded sizes of print.

A small child (or illiterate) can be tested by asking him to match the graded Snellen letters of the distant chart with a set of similar letters held

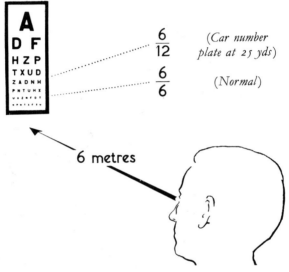

Fig. 1.5. Testing visual acuity by Snellen's types.

in his hand (the 'Sheridan–Gardiner test'), or to place his hand in the position of a series of hands (of graded sizes) painted on cards held by the examiner. In infants, the fixation of light or of moving fingers, and the pupil response will give some indication of the visual acuity.

Visual fields

The visual fields can be quickly assessed by the confrontation test, in which the patient closes one eye, looking straight with the other eye into the corresponding eye of the surgeon, and signals as soon as he can see the surgeon's fingers which are introduced in turn from the periphery on the four diagonal positions. A more exact record is offered by the perimeter (Fig. 1.6) which charts the position where a small white target first becomes visible in each successive meridian, while the patient keeps his uncovered eye fixed on the 'hub' of the instrument (cf. charts, Figs. 4.9, 9.2, 9.4, 9.5).

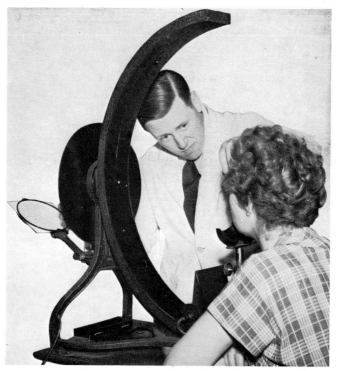

Fig. 1.6. Technique of perimetry, with the self-recording perimeter. (Blaxter.)

Colour-blindness

Colour-blindness is a curious hereditary defect found in about 8 per cent of men and 0·4 per cent of women, usually entailing a difficulty in differentiating red and green; it is readily tested by presenting a series of book-plates in which the different coloured spots spell out a number which will be specifically misinterpreted by the various colour-blind variants. **Night-blindness** is another hereditary defect, less readily tested, equally important in certain employments, and equally untreatable.

Infants

In infants and the very retarded, examination of the eye ('veterinary ophthalmology') may require firm measures; the child should be wrapped tightly in a blanket, laid on a couch, with its head rigidly held between the assistant's hands, and its body pinioned between the assistant's elbows. The eyelids can then be prised apart by simple 'retractors'. If the fundus also needs inspection, the wandering eye may have to be secured by conjunctival forceps after local or general anaesthesia.

CHAPTER 2
THE EYELIDS, LACRIMAL APPARATUS AND ORBIT

The eyelids are protective folds, covered by skin on the outside and a thin layer of conjunctiva beneath, (this is the 'tarsal conjunctiva', as opposed to 'bulbar conjunctiva' where this same layer is continued over the surface of the sclera, and 'fornix conjunctiva', which unites these two in the recesses of the 'conjunctival sac'). The substance of the eyelid consists of two layers; anteriorly the Orbicularis Oculi muscle which closes the lid, and posteriorly a tarsal plate, the thickened wall of a row of 20–30 elongated sebaceous ('Meibomian') glands, which serves as a skeleton to the lid. Between these two layers lie the terminal fibres of the Levator Palpebrae Superioris muscle (Fig. 2.1).

The eyelid margin is divided longitudinally by a grey line, marking the junction of skin and conjunctiva; along the anterior strip lie the eyelashes with sudorific and sebaceous glands at their roots, and behind these lie the openings of the Meibomian glands (just visible to the naked eye).

CONGENITAL MALFORMATIONS

Ptosis (a droop of the upper lid) calls for surgical correction if it is too unsightly, or in more extreme cases if it covers the pupil and interferes with vision; as ptosis is usually bilateral, such children may have to tilt their heads backwards in order to see beneath the drooping lids. Many operations have been proposed, but it is usually best simply to resect some of the levator palpebrae superioris muscle and of the upper tarsal plate.

Ptosis may also follow damage to the lid, levator muscle or its motor innervation (as in myasthenia gravis or tabes), or as a senile myasthenia when the lax tissues of old-age tend to sag.

Epicanthic folds are vertical pleats of skin between the medial ends of the upper and lower lids which tend to overlap the medial angle of the eye (Fig. 2.2). These are common in infants, where they often give the illusion of a convergent squint, and disappear when the nasal bones grow; occasionally they persist and require operative correction; and they are a normal feature of mongoloid races and 'mongolian' idiots.

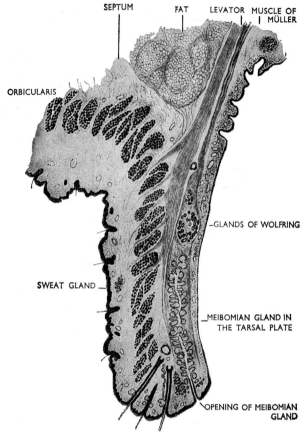

Fig. 2.1. Vertical section through the upper lid. (Wolff, *Anatomy of the Eye and Orbit.*)

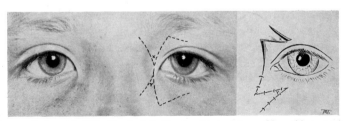

Fig. 2.2. Epicanthic folds. On the left side, the skin incisions of Spaeth's operation are marked, and the triangular flaps are rotated as in the diagram alongside.

INFLAMMATION OF THE EYELIDS

Styes are localized infections of the glands of the lid margin. The more common 'external stye' (or 'Hordeolum'—Fig. 2.3) is a simple pyogenic infection of one of the glands at the lash-base, analogous to furuncles elsewhere; after a few days of painful induration, it normally discharges its bead of pus, and is gone. No treatment is necessary; heat is a mild palliative and doubtful expediter, and antibiotic ointment may prevent the emergent staphylococci from infecting another lash follicle farther down the line.

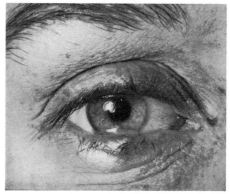

Fig. 2.3. External stye

The 'internal stye' is a similar infection of one of the Meibomian glands. Since the gland-wall is tough, the pus rarely bursts through the skin or conjunctival surface, so that the inflammation is brought under control more slowly; and since the outlet of the gland has normally become blocked, its secretion combined with the inflammatory exudate distend the gland, leaving a residual cyst— a meibomian cyst—(Fig. 2.4), also known as 'Chalazion', since it fells like a hailstone embedded in the tarsal plate. These cysts are usually symptomless and may even develop insidiously, but, once established, they can be dispersed by incising vertically through the conjunctival surface and evacuating their mucinous content with a curette (Fig. 2.5).

A blepharitis is a generalized infection of the margins of the eyelids, making the lid-margins look red, with a variable itchiness and an occasional discharge. This infection is notoriously persistent, and after some years the lashes may fall out, or by turning inwards irritate and ulcerate the

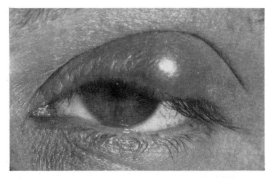

Fig. 2.4. Meibomian cyst.

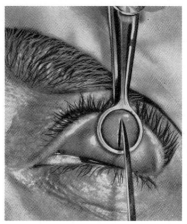

Fig. 2.5. Evacuation of meibomian cyst.

cornea. The milder form of blepharitis—'squamous blepharitis'—is essentially an outpost of dandruff from the scalp in seborrhoeic subjects, exhibiting similar scales clinging to the lashes, and provoking a similar variable irritation. The more severe 'ulcerative blepharitis' (Fig. 2.6) involves a staphylococcal infection on top of the seborrhoeic inflammation, and the lid margins become manifestly indurated and even ulcerated. Treatment must be long-sustained to be effective, as the infection is hard to eradicate. It entails (1) control of the scalp infection by frequent shampoos and anti-dandruff inunctions; (2) removal of all crusts and discharge from the lashes by an alkaline lotion, trimming the lashes if necessary; (3) drops or ointment containing a hydrocortisone and an antibiotic (as neomycin or chloramphenicol) to the lid margins, using these as often as the symptoms demand them (hourly, if necessary) and resorting to them at every relapse.

A seborrhoic blepharitis is probably the commonest cause of all chronic eye discomforts, and it can nearly always be allayed simply by the use of topical steroids; but these must be prescribed with caution, as they carry the risk of exacerbating a dendritic corneal ulcer, or promoting a simple glaucoma (although the latter is rare before middle-age).

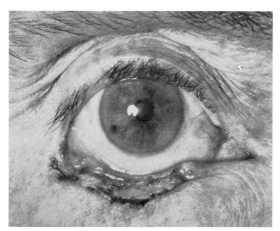

Fig. 2.6. Ulcerative blepharitis.

DISPLACEMENTS OF THE EYELIDS

The eyelids may become everted or inverted, and this may be due to *spasm* or *atony* of the orbicularis; or from *scarring*, which everts if the skin is scarred—a 'cicatricial ectropion', as after burns of the face, and inverts if the tarsal conjunctiva is scarred—a 'cicatricial entropion', as in trachoma (Fig. 3.3). The common adult forms affect the less rigid lower lids, causing a spastic entropion or an atonic ectropion.

Spastic entropion (Fig. 2.7) is the product of persistent screwing-up and rubbing of the eyes, in irritable old people with irritable conjunctivas. A vicious circle develops, the lashes becoming inturned and causing more corneal and conjunctival irritation, with still further stimulus to entropion. Lubricants and sedatives may relieve, but surgery is usually needed. In this the bundle of orbicularis fibres nearest to the lower lid margin is

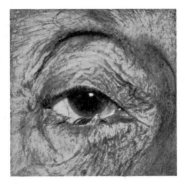

Fig. 2.7. Spastic entropion.

drawn laterally and tethered to the temporal fascia; or else it is simply
excised along with an overlying strip of skin (a 'skin-and-muscle operation').

Atonic ectropion (Fig. 2.8) may be due to a flaccid orbicularis from a
facial nerve palsy, or more commonly just a senile loss of tone of the lower
lid muscles, which lets the lid droop away from the eyeball. A vicious circle
again develops, since a stagnant pool of tears forms in the lower fornix,
becomes infected, and causes a thickening of the inflamed conjunctiva
which mechanically pushes the lid farther away, and increases the epiphora (= weeping) which is the main complaint. Astringents may reduce
the epiphora and antibiotics may reduce the infection, but an operation is
again usually necessary, either to improve the lacrimal drainage by enlarg-

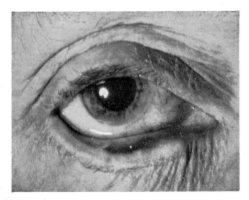

Fig. 2.8. Atonic ectropion.

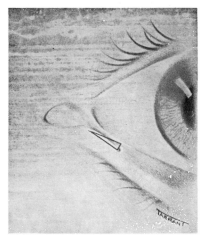

Fig. 2.9. Incisions for the Three-snip operation.

ing the punctum backwards into the stagnant pool (a'three-snip operation'—Fig. 2.9), or as a plastic operation to tauten the lid.

TUMOURS AND DEGENERATIONS

Among benign tumours of the lids the most singular are Xanthelasmata, which are intradermal plaques of creamy xanthomatous deposits, generally sysmmetrical, and sited at the medial ends of the upper or lower lids (Fig. 2.10). They are rarely related to any generalized lipoidosis, although they tend to arise in women of 'gallstone' diathesis; and they can always be excised if disfiguring. Papillomata are fairly common where conjunctiva and skin meet at the lid-margin, and may grow into horns several inches long. Dermoid cysts arise classically at the upper inner and outer angles of the orbit, while creamy 'dermolipomata' are sometimes found astride the infant's corneo-scleral margin.

Of malignant tumours, **rodent ulcers** frequently arise (and carcinomas occasionally) at the lid-margin, and should be excised, or, if this would render plastic repair too clumsy, irradiated. **Carcinoma of the lacrimal gland** is much rarer, resembling in its structure and behaviour a mixed parotid tumour, since it generally starts as a benign adenoma, which, being loculated, is not easily removed completely; and recurrences often become malignant. In such cases it may be necessary to excavate the entire orbital contents (an 'exenteration').

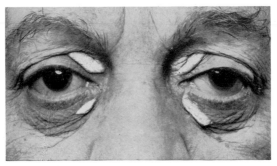

Fig. 2.10. Xanthelasma.

Pingueculae and **Pterygia** are fairly common degenerative growths on the front of the eye, which may be included here. A Pinguecula (Plate 3, following p. 60) is a fatty deposit under the conjunctiva which is often most arresting when it fails to share in any coincident conjunctival congestion; a Pterygium is a wing-shaped fold of conjunctiva that gradually transgresses onto the cornea, and may even reach the central area and impair vision (Fig. 2.11). Both are symptomless and symmetrical, involve only the medial and lateral sides, and tend to occur after a life of exposure to the elements; and both of them can readily be excised, although the resultant scar may yield little cosmetic improvement. The Pterygium may also need excision if it threatens the sight, and various techniques are employed to try to prevent recurrence. Other purely corneal degenerations include the familar **arcus senilis** (a white encircling ring, about 1 mm within the corneal margin) which affects only the periphery, and therefore never

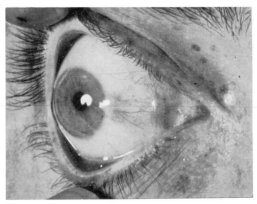

Fig. 2.11. Pterygium.

damages sight; and the **familial dystrophies**. which affect the central area, and distort the vision. The latter can readily be remedied by a corneal graft (p. 46, Fig 3.17).

LACRIMAL DISORDERS

The *tears*, which moisten, lave and disinfect the surface of the eye, are secreted by the lacrimal gland which lies beneath the overhanging superolateral orbital rim. They are drained away through two lacrimal 'puncta' at the inner end of the lid margins, leading via two narrow canaliculi into the lacrimal sac; this lies in a fossa in the lacrimal bone, collects the tears from the two canaliculi and transmits them downwards through the nasolacrimal duct into the lower meatus of the nasal cavity (Fig. 2.12).

A *dry* eye is the sequel to undersecretion, which mainly occurs in older women when the lacrimal and parotid glands become sclerosed ('Sjogren's Syndrome', or 'Keratoconjunctivitis Sicca'). This dryness, along with the pain from the secondary corneal erosions, may be allayed by instilling 'artificial tears'.

A *wet* eye usually stems from a blockage to the exit channels; an overflow of tears ('epiphora') may thus be the legacy of a block at the

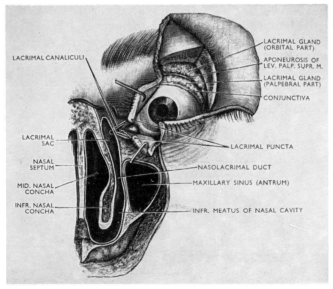

Fig. 2.12. The anatomy of the lacrimal apparatus. (Gray's *Anatomy*.)

punctum (sometimes it is plugged by a detached eye-lash,), or in the canaliculus (as from a laceration of the lid margin or by cheesy agglomerations of streptothrix), or else simply by an eversion of the lid margin (ectropion). More usually it follows an obstruction of the nasolacrimal duct, either as a result of a sac infection (dacryocystitis), or in the infant from a failure in canalization (in which case a secondary dacryocystitis soon follows).

Acute dacryocystitis usually follows an infection which ascends from the nasopharynx, and it is evidenced by a tender induration at the medial angle of the eye. Pus may rupture through the skin forming a fistula, but more usually it resolves (especially when allayed by local heat and systemic antibiotics), to leave a *chronic dacryocystitis* with a blocked nasolacrimal duct, and sometimes a visibly distended 'mucocele' of the sac; more often a chronic dacryocystitis develops without antecedent acute phase, particularly in elderly women. The only symptom of chronic dacryocystitis is epiphora, and the overflowing tears may be augmented by the discharge from a chronic conjunctivitis (which has been provoked by the regurgitation of pus along the lacrimal canaliculi).

The treatment of such a watering eye first entails syringing of saline through the lower canaliculus (Fig. 2.13); this shows whether there is a nasolacrimal duct obstruction, and in the early stages may in fact clear the blocked passage. This can be followed by astringent drops or lotions, such as Zinc Sulphate $\frac{1}{4}$ per cent, to reduce the watering. If the epiphora is sufficiently troublesome and has not yielded to several syringings, an operation may be justified; this should be a 'dacryocysto-rhinostomy' (Fig. 2.14), fashioning a new stoma between the sac and the underlying middle

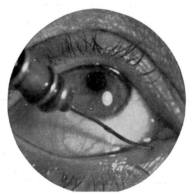

Fig. 2.13. Syringing the lacrimal sac.

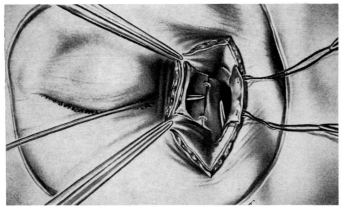

Fig. 2.14. Dacryocystorhinostomy. The posterior flaps of the medial sac wall and nasal mucosa have been sutured together. Probes have been inserted through the canaliculus and the nose, to demonstrate the reconstituted passage. (Lyle.)

meatus of the nasopharynx; however in the old and debile, especially where regurgitation of pus is the main trouble, a 'dacryocystetomy' may suffice to ease the symptoms by simply removing the source of conjunctival re-infection. Probing the nasolacrimal duct is of value only in the absence of established infection, as when the duct has failed to canalize in infants. Such cases are usually cured by toiled and antibiotic drops alone, but probing is generally advised if the blockage persists for several months. Finally, epiphora may be relieved, when the lacrimal outlet cannot be re-established, by reducing the production of tears, either by excising or by injecting alcohol into the lacrimal gland (at the outer, upper angle of the orbit).

EXOPHTHALMOS

Any lesion within the unyielding bony walls of the orbit tends to push the eyeball forwards and present as an exophthalmos (or 'proptosis', which strictly means a protrusion of the lids as well). Where the pressure is exerted from directly behind the eye (as from a haemorrhage, inflammation or tumour within the cone of the four rectus muscles) the eye is pushed directly forwards; but an eccentric pressure (as from a periostitis, orbital fracture or lacrimal gland tumour) will deviate the eyeball, and usually cause diplopia, unless the sight has already been destroyed.

Carotico-cavernous fistula

Damage to the carotid artery from trauma or spontaneous rupture of a carotid aneurysm within the enveloping cavernous sinus, may lead to a carotico-cavernous fistula, with a reflux of arterial blood under pressure into the orbital veins. It presents classically as a 'pulsating exophthalmos', and though the systolic pulsations may be barely visible, they are audible both to the auscultating surgeon and to the patient as an alarming noise, likened to the buzz of a bluebottle within a paper bag or the rush of a millstream. The conjunctival vessels are visibly engorged, and both lids and conjunctivae may be very oedematous; these same signs are usually present, but less well-marked, on the other eye (because of the connecting intercavernous sinuses). The condition is generally stationary, but the initial pain recedes, and in the absence of ocular complications the impaired vision may also slowly improve. Radical treatment entails ligation of the common carotid or (if this fails) internal carotid artery, both yielding about a 50 per cent cure and an appreciable mortality rate.

Orbital cellulitis (Fig. 2.15)

Orbital cellulitis, generally deriving from an adjacent sinusitis, is fairly common, and grave, because of the risk of damage to the eye or of extension back to the meninges. The eyeball protrudes and becomes immobile, and the sight may be extinguished by pressure on the optic nerve (although a pallor of the optic disc will not be visible for some weeks, and the fundus at first shows only a venous engorgement); pain is often severe until pus is evacuated, but prompt treatment with systemic antibiotics usually permits resolution without any recourse to operative drainage.

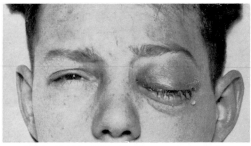

Fig. 2.15. Acute orbital cellulitis, following an acute sinusitis, and exhibiting proptosis with oedema of lids and conjunctiva.

Cavernous sinus thrombosis

This thrombosis may be the drastic sequel to orbital cellulitis or may follow some simple pyogenic infection such as a furuncle that has drained via the angular vein into the cavernous sinus. The signs and symptoms are largely an aggravation of those of an orbital cellulitis, but the degree of pain, extreme venous congestion and bilaterality are usually diagnostic; in any event the same treatment obtains, supplemented by anticoagulants to prevent extensions of the septic clot.

Dysthyroid exophthalmos

There are two main types of ophthalmic manifestation in thyroid disease, mild and severe, the one merging imperceptibly into the other.

The mild type (Fig. 2.16) occurs classically in patients with Graves' disease and is seen most commonly in women aged 20–50, along with the general signs of thyrotoxicosis (tremor, sweating, wasting and tachycardia). Lid-retraction and lid-lag are often marked and result in a prominent stare; there may, in addition, be a mild degree of proptosis. The systemic treatment is that of the underlying hyperthyroidism, and includes sedatives, antithyroid drugs, radio-active iodine and thyroidectomy. The ocular changes rarely merit attention, but a small lateral tarsorrhaphy may be cosmetically helpful, while lid retraction sometimes responds to guanethidine eye-drops, indicating its probable origin from overactivity of the sympathetic nervous system.

The severe type (Fig. 2.17) is much less common and affects the sexes equally, at an average age of 50. It often follows the treatment of hyperthyroidism and the patient may show under- or over-activity of the gland. This condition is not clearly understood but it is apparently caused by an exophthalmos-producing substance, probably a gamma globulin and possibly a product of the pituitary gland. The systemic signs are usually slight and the ocular signs predominate, with a gross and irreducible exophthalmos, frequently leading to corneal ulceration, a marked ophthalmoplegia especially of upward movement and even preceding the exophthalmos, and a marked oedema of lids and conjunctivae. These changes are due to an infiltration and oedema with subsequent fibrosis of the muscles themselves, and to a lesser extent of the other orbital tissues. Systemic treatment of the underlying thyroid condition is neither very efficacious nor very necessary since the condition is self-limiting, but the grave risk of corneal damage or strangulation of the optic nerve generally calls for

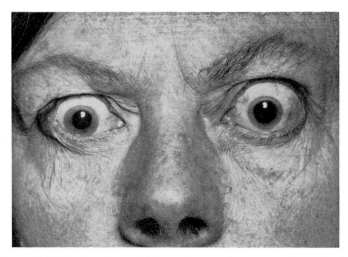

Fig. 2.16. Mild dysthyroid exophthalmos (Graves's disease); lateral tarsorrhaphy has been performed on the R. side.

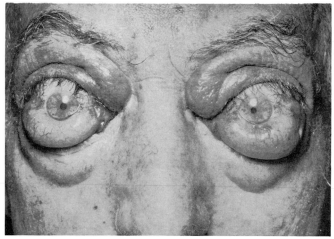

Fig. 2.17. Severe dysthyroid exophthalmos; with ophthalmoplegia and oedema.

urgent treatment. Some cases respond dramatically to large doses of systemic steroids, but failing this a wide tarsorrhaphy or even an orbital decompression may be necessary.

Orbital tumours

Either primary (meningioma or glioma of optic nerve), secondary to spread from adjacent sinuses (carcinoma of antrum may present by obstructing the tear duct, just as frontal or ethmoidal mucoceles often cause proptosis), or metastases (especially in children, from leukaemia, neuroblastoma, Wilm's tumour).

CHAPTER 3
THE PAINFUL RED EYE

There are three main causes of the painful red eye: inflammation of the outer eye (acute **conjunctivitis**), inflammation of the inner eye (**acute iritis**), and the congested, tense eyeball due to a sudden blockage of aqueous outflow (**acute glaucoma**). A knowledge of their differential diagnosis is consequently of extreme importance since the majority of eye affections demanding urgent treatment fall into one of these three categories. A fourth major cause of painful red eyes should properly be added to this list—an **acute keratitis**, which generally presents as the familiar 'corneal ulcer'; and of this (since the cornea is the gateway between the outer and inner eyes), the symptoms, signs and treatment tend to be a combination of those of an acute conjunctivitis and an acute iritis.

ACUTE CONJUNCTIVITIS

SIGNS AND SYMPTOMS

1. *The eye is red*—this is due to a generalized dilatation of the surface vessels, a 'conjunctival injection'; it is equally manifest in the tarsal conjunctiva which lines the posterior surface of the eyelids (in contrast to the purely 'circumcorneal injection' of acute iritis and acute glaucoma) (Fig. 3.1).
2. *Discharge*—this may be purulent, mucopurulent or catarrhal, according to severity of infection; it is most noticeable on waking, when the lids are often glued together.
3. *Discomfort*—this is a grittiness rather than a pain, primarily caused by the rubbing together of congested bulbar and lid conjunctivae with every movement of the eyelids.
4. *Photophobia*—this is so mild that it can be relieved by dark glasses.

AETIOLOGICAL TYPES

The common catarrhal conjunctivitis is usually due to *Staph. aureus*; the

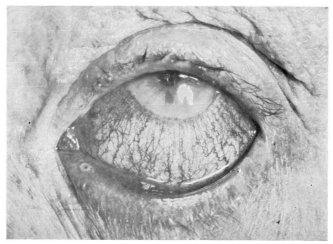

Fig. 3.1. Acute infective conjunctivitis, with slight secondary ectropion and pouting of the lacrimal punctum.

rarer severe bout may be due to *Pneumococcus*. Less common types include 'Epidemic pink-eye' due to *Haemophilus influenzae*. The healthy conjunctiva often harbours *Straphylococcus albus* and *Corynebacterium xerosis*.

Most forms of acute conjunctivitis essentially resemble a nasal catarrh, subside within a week without lasting damage, and may be allayed by treatment. More serious (especially in tropical and sub-tropical countries) are the conjunctival infections due to the gonococcus ('ophthalmia neonatorum') and chlamydia ('inclusion conjunctivitis').

Ophthalmia neonatorum

Severe purulent conjunctivitis, (Fig. 3.2) contracted at birth from a *gonococcal* infection of the maternal passages. Formerly a cause of widespread blindness (from secondary corneal ulceration), it became rare after the general adoption of Crédé's prophylactic drops of 1–2 per cent silver nitrate; nowadays these drops can safely be omitted, as long as subsequent medical supervision is ensured (for once recognized, gonococcal conjunctivitis now yields promptly to intensive penicillin application or sulphonamides by mouth). Any eye discharge within 3 weeks of birth is a notifiable disease, although such a discharge is generally due to a chlamydial infection, and free from danger.

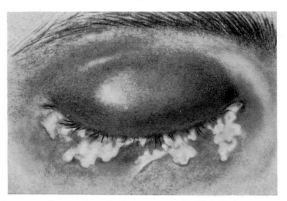

Fig. 3.2. Acute purulent conjunctivitis (gonococcal 'ophthalmia neonatorum').

Inclusion conjunctivitis

Certain forms of acute conjunctivitis can be differentiated by the presence of basophil cytoplasmic inclusion bodies within the epithelial cells. These are composed of organisms ('elementary bodies') 0·25–0·4 μm in size, which are liberated when the cell bursts and then infect another cell.

The organism responsible for the various clinical manifestations of Inclusion conjunctivitis is known as the TRIC agent, and belongs to the genus *Chlamydia*, along with the other atypical viruses of the PLT (Psittacosis, lymphogranuloma vernereum, trachoma) group; these lie midway between true viruses and bacteria, are filterable yet divide by binary fission, have both DNA and RNA and a complex struture approaching that of bacteria.

In the eye, the TRIC agent can present with four different clinical patterns: trachoma, simple inclusion conjunctivitis of adult or newborn, and a kerato-conjunctivitis; and although these separate manifestations may appear at different stages in the same individual, or in different members of the same household, they are sufficiently distinctive to merit separate discussion.

Trachoma is a disease of world-wide distribution, whose ravages are written across history; and even today affects about a fifth of the world's inhabitants, and is overall the commonest cause of blindness from scarring of the cornea. Initially this scarring follows a direct infection of the cornea, but it is also provoked in the later stages, when cicatrization of the tarsal plate has induced an ectropion (leading to a neurotrophic keratitis from exposure) or an entropion (with inturned lashes abrading the cornea) (Fig.

3.3, and see p. 17). Lymphoid hyperplasia is a characteristic of most viral conjunctivites, and the resultant follicles, about 2 mm wide, are especially apparent in trachoma, where they may cover the under surfaces of the tarsal plates (Fig. 3.4). Trachoma has been endemic since pre-history in the Middle East, and sporadic in most other countries of the world with the striking and almost universal exception of the British Commonwealth; devastating outbreaks have followed in the wake of most invading armies that reached the Middle East (Crusades, Napoleonic wars) or set out from there (Mohammedan invasions). The chlamydium is just within the range of antibiotic and sulphonamide therapy, which will also control any secondary bacterial infection. Vaccines are available; but the essential

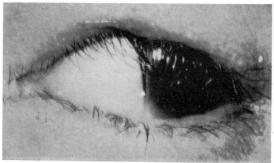

Fig. 3.3. Late trachoma. Cicatricial entropion of the upper lid with inturned lashes. (Scheie.)

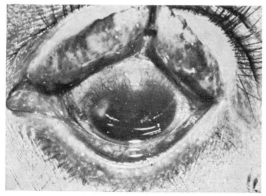

Fig. 3.4. Early trachoma. The upper tarsal conjunctiva is grossly thickened and covered in follicles, while a vascularized infiltrate ('pannus') is extending down over the upper cornea. (Scheie.)

treatment consists in avoiding reinfection. In Western cultures—more hygienic but more promiscuous—the TRIC chlamydium is a common infector of the genital tract. The cicatricial entropion that is the usual cause of blindness can be rectified by a variety of quite simple plastic operations that evert the inturned upper lid-margin with its ingrowing lashes.

Epidemic kerato-conjunctivitis occurs sporadically in England, but as widespread outbreaks in tropical countries. It presents with an oedematous conjunctiva (developing follicles on its tarsal surface), and tiny spots on the cornea ('superficial punctate keratitis') often associated with pharyngitis and pre-auricular lymphadenopathy. It is caused by adenovirus type 8, which, unlike the agent of trachoma, is outside the range of sulpha and antibiotic drugs; atropine and a pad normally allow resolution in about two weeks, otherwise the corneal infiltrate may spread and damage the sight, especially if topical steroids are used.

ALLERGIC CONJUNCTIVITIS

The conjunctiva often becomes hypersensitive to a miscellany of irritants. Some of these, such as the drugs (especially atropine and penicillin) or the cosmetics with which it is belaboured, principally affect the eyelids, causing eczema and oedema (Fig. 3.5). Other exogenous allergens, such as pollens, cause an extreme congestion and watering of the conjunctival and

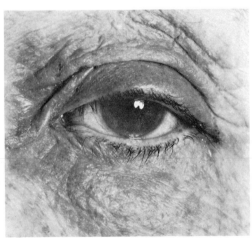

Fig. 3.5. 'Atropine irritation,' Allergic dermato-conjunctivitis due to atropine-sensitivity.

nasal mucosa, as in **hay fever**. Allergy from pollens may also be chronic and seasonal, as in **Spring catarrh**, characterized by flat-topped, translucent papules, mainly over the tarsal conjunctiva (Fig. 3.6).

Endogenous allergens, such as tuberculo-protein, may provoke a **phlyctenular conjunctivitis** in poorly nourished children but now rarely seen. This is characterized by subconjunctival aggregations of lymphocytes ('phlyctens'), which contrast with the surrounding engorgement; they occasionally transgress onto the cornea (Fig. 3.7).

Conjunctival allergies usually respond specifically to treatment with

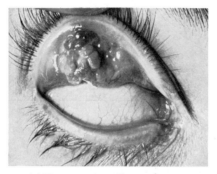

Fig. 3.6. 'Spring catarrh.' Flat-topped papillae on the upper tarsal conjunctiva.

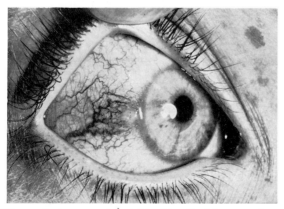

Fig. 3.7. Phlyctenular kerato-conjunctivitis with yellowish aggregations of leucocytes on the conjunctiva and encroaching onto the cornea.

drops of corticosteroids or anti-histamines (as Otrivine–Antistin), and can generally be allayed by astringents; desensitization is rarely applicable.

TREATMENT OF CONJUNCTIVITIS

1. *Remove any discharge by simple toilet with a moist swab.* If there is copious discharge, irrigation is necessary and may be comforting (Fig. 3.8).

2. *Bactericidal applications.* These must be given every hour or two to be of value. Chloramphenicol and neomycin have a wide antibiotic spectrum, are stable and relatively cheap. For resistant strains, other antibiotic drops are indicated such as gentamycin and polymyxin. Topical sulphonamides are rarely indicated, but sulphacetamide ('Albucid') is popular and of limited value.

3. *Symptomatic treatment.* Dark-glasses will allay the mild photophobia, but an eye-pad should be avoided since it may retain the discharge and

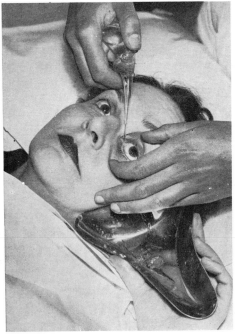

Fig. 3.8. Irrigation of the conjunctiva with an undine.

incubate the pathogens. Lubricant drops as hypromellose (1 per cent) may relieve the 'grittiness', or the lubricant may be provided in the form of an ointment vehicle for the antibiotic agent.

4.   *Astringent applications.* Solutions of metallic salts will decongest and dry an inflamed eye, and relieve the feeling of heaviness and irritability. They are particularly useful where in flammation is due to allergy, external irritants (smoke, ultra-violet light, etc.), or when the eye remains red after infection has been cleared by antibiotic treatment. Zinc sulphate ($\frac{1}{4}$ per cent drops or lotion) or silver proteinate drops are traditional; but where there is an allergic factor, corticosteroid drops are most effective (although to be used with caution—see p. 15).

ACUTE IRITIS

The iris, ciliary body and choroid form a continuous sheet along the inner wall of corneo-sclera, known as the 'uveal tract' and although each component is to some extent involved in any intra-ocular inflammation, the clinical picture of uveitis varies with the main site of its impact. When the burden falls on the anterior uvea (an 'iritis' or an 'irido-cyclitis') the eye becomes *painful* from oedema and from spasm of the iris and ciliary muscles, and *red* from engorgement of the adjacent circumcorneal vessels which are connected through the sclera with the vessels of the iris root. A 'choroiditis' is correspondingly painless, free from any visible congestion on the front of the eye, and presents simply with an *impaired vision* (p. 58).

SIGNS AND SYMPTOMS

1.   Engorgement of the episcleral vessels overlying the iris root, as a 'ciliary' or **'circumcorneal injection'** (Plate 4, following p. 48). This differs from a 'conjunctival injection' (in which vessels are engorged evenly over the whole conjunctival surface—'tarsal' as well as 'bulbar') qualitatively as well as geographically, since these deeper episcleral vessels seem less discrete through the overlying conjunctiva (the term 'ciliary flush' is thus sometimes used), and the colour is brick-red rather than pink (it becomes purple when a venous stasis rather than an inflammatory injection is responsible, as in the ciliary injection of an acute glaucoma).

2.   **Contraction of the pupil**, to which reflex spasm of the sphincter and the distension of the iris with blood both contribute.

3.   Inflammatory **exudation** into the anterior chamber. Pus cells can

always be discerned with the corneal microscope as a pathognominic sign, and these may be so profuse that they gravitate to form an obvious fluid-level at the bottom of the anterior chamber, known as a **hypopyon** (Figs. 3.13 and 3.15). They also adhere to the back of the cornea froming clumps which are often visible macroscopically, and known as **keratic precipitates,** or more familiarly 'K.P.' (Fig. 3.9). This exudate causes a proportionate **blurring of vision,** especially when it also passes from the ciliary body into the vitreous (whence it is less readily dispersed).

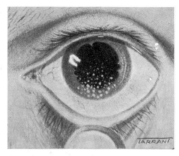

Fig. 3.9. Keratic precipitates.

4.   Adhesions between iris and the anterior lens surface, with which it is normally in contact. These are known as **'posterior synechias',** as opposed to the rare 'anterior synechias' between iris and cornea, which may follow an escape of aqueous through a perforating corneal wound or ulcer. Such posterior synechias are often rendered obvious when the therapeutic atropine drops cause a festooning of the pupil, since this can dilate only between those points where its margin is already bound-down to the lens (Plate 4, following p. 60 and Fig. 3.9). Should the whole pupillary margin become adherent, the aqueous, which diffuses from the anterior surface of the iris and the ciliary body, cannot pass forwards through the pupil to reach its exit into the canal of Schlemm; and the iris may then become ballooned forward (an 'iris bombé'), and the intra-ocular pressure will rise (a 'secondary glaucoma').

5.   The eyeball is **tender** and **painful**; this pain is constant, and does not cease when the eyelids are stilled, and may thus keep the patient awake at night, unlike the simple irritation provoked by a conjunctivitis.

6.   Photophobia. Light seems positively hurtful to the eye, unlike the mild light-sensitivity from a conjunctivitis which dark glasses will normally allay, and the lids may be difficult to open ('blepharospasm'); this is generally accompanied by a little reflex lacrimation (unlike the manifest inflammatory discharge of an acute conjunctivitis).

Acute iritis tends to last for weeks or even months, relapses being common, and leaving some permanent visual damage if uncontrolled. Sometimes the iritis is chronic, with little pain and injection, but the sight is insidiously reduced by the exudate, especially when this permeates behind the lens into the vitreous cavity. Complications include: **secondary glaucoma**, where exudate or adhesions impede drainage of the aqueous, and **secondary cataract** through impairment of lens nutrition.

AETIOLOGICAL TYPES OF ACUTE IRITIS

Iritis (and uveitis generally) is occasionally caused by *exogenous* infection, gaining admission through perforating wounds of the eyeball or corneal ulcers, and leading to a purulent 'endophthalmitis', which becomes a 'panophthalmitis' if the outer coats have been invaded.

The large majority of cases of iritis are *endogenous*, and the cause is generally unknown; over the last fifty years these have been attributed in turn to syphilis, tuberculosis, focal sepsis (especially teeth), allergy, virus disease, auto-immunity and metabolic upset. A small percentage seem indeed to be due to each of these groups, as well as a variety of other affections (as brucellosis, sarcoidosis, toxoplasmosis, gonorrhoea); but the majority, whose cause remains obscure, probably stem from an auto-antibody reaction, and are often associated with ankylosing spondylitis. In investigating such cases, it is thus usual to exclude a positive Wassermann reaction, radiographic evidence of spondylitis or of infective foci in teeth, sinuses and chest, and possibly perform a Mantoux test, toxoplasmosis test and blood analysis.

Sympathetic ophthalmitis is a specific form of iritis (or, more correctly, of uveitis), which generally follows perforating wounds near the corneo-scleral junction, including operations as for cataract, and which involves the other eye some weeks later, and is so persistent that it may render both eyes almost blind. It very rarely occurs within ten days after the initiating injury, but any traumatic iritis which is not subsiding after such an interval is dangerous, and such an eye may even require excision to prevent the risk of involving its fellow. In treatment, corticosteroids are of especial benefit.

TREATMENT OF ACUTE IRITIS

1. **Corticosteroids**, which simply inhibit the inflammatory response, are of enormous value in allaying any uveitis, except in the very rare case where there is a frank infective agent, for most uveites are essentially self-limiting, and both the ultimate damage and the degree of pain that is provoked are largely proportional to the intensity of the inflammatory reaction. Patients with this form of anterior uveitis should receive as much steroid as is necessary to keep the eye quiet. Topical application is of course free of any systemic side-effects as well as the expense of systemic steroid therapy, so drops or ointment ($\frac{1}{4}$ per cent) are normally prescribed for insertion into the conjunctival sac, every hour if necessary. If this does not suffice to suppress the aqueous exudate, prednisolone can be injected subconjunctivally, and given systemically (as tablets, 5 mg. up to six times a day).

2. **Atropine**, which paralyses the ciliary muscle and iris sphincter, allows physiological rest and relief from the pain due to spasm; it also encourages the blood-flow, and dilates the pupil so that any posterior synechias will be formed well away from the central (visual) area. One per cent atropine sulphate drops or ointment are normally given 2–3 times a day, reducing to $\frac{1}{2}$ per cent daily as the inflammation wanes. Atropine-sensitivity frequently develops, especially when the stronger concentrations are used, leading to eczema of the lids and conjunctiva (Fig. 3.5); in such cases many weaker substitutes are available, particularly hyoscine; homatropine causes only a transient pupillary dilatation and a negligible ciliary paresis, so that it is rarely used except as a diagnostic aid in ophthalmoscopy and retinoscopy. These mydriatics, by forcibly dilating the pupil, may very exceptionally provoke an acute glaucoma in eyes that happen to have very shallow anterior chambers; so, after inducing a mydriasis for ophthalmoscopy, it is wise to constrict the pupil again with a drop of eserine.

3. **Heat** (as from an electric pad or hot fomentation) will relieve the pain and allay the inflammation.

4. A **pad**, which keeps the lid firmly closed over the eye, will provide rest and relieve photophobia.

Any underlying disease should be sought and treated; the patient should rest, and any complication of the iritis may require specific measures (e.g. a secondary glaucoma will need acetazolamide, and surgical drainage if uncontrolled).

ACUTE GLAUCOMA

Glaucoma signifies an increased intra-ocular pressure. The term was originally coined because of the grey-green colour (as of a stormy sea) that the waterlogged cornea transmits in an acute glaucoma, and it was later applied to the insidious chronic form now known as 'simple glaucoma', which was also characterized by a raised intra-ocular pressure but in which the front of the eye looked normal. Both acute and simple glaucoma may be *secondary* to a manifest and specific eye disease which interferes with aqueous drainage (as iritis, or an intra-ocular tumour), but for the majority of cases no overt cause is apparent and these are labelled *primary*. Both acute and chronic glaucoma are rare before middle-age.

Primary acute glaucoma (or, more properly, 'closed-angle' glaucoma) is characterized by bouts of raised tension. These are largely precipitated by a protrusion of the iris root, so that it makes contact with the back of the cornea, shuts off the peripheral recess of the anterior chamber, and thus prevents aqueous escaping into the canal of Schlemm. Attacks are thus virtually confined to eyes with a very shallow anterior chamber, and consequently a very narrow drainage-angle. This protrusion is usually caused by damming-up of aqueous behind the iris, since in mid-dilatation of the pupil the area of lens–iris contact is greatest, and forward passage of aqueous through the pupil is then impeded (Fig. 3.10). It is aggravated by the natural thickening of the iris root that accompanies pupillary dila-

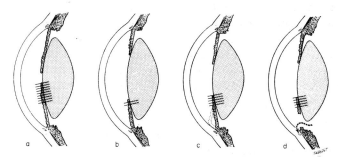

Fig. 3.10. Mechanism of angle-closure glaucoma. (*a*) When pupil constricted, although large area of lens-iris contact, the iris is taut and does not balloon forwards. (*b*) When pupil dilated, although iris lax, aqueous readily escapes through pupil as small area of lens-iris contact. (*c*) When pupil mid-dilated, larger area of lens-iris contact impedes escape of aqueous through pupil, and aqueous presses relatively lax iris root forwards to block drainage-angle, unless aqueous is enabled to escape freely through a peripheral iridectomy as in (*d*).

tation, perhaps abetted by vasodilatation and oedema. Such acute glau-
comas are more common in the middle-aged, and occur especially in
hypermetropes (the smaller eyeball having a proportionately shallower
anterior chamber); the attacks themselves are often precipitated when
emotion or fading light causes the pupil to dilate.

steamy cornea
oedematous iris
congested ciliary body

SIGNS AND SYMPTOMS

The acute glaucoma usually starts with severe pain in, and radiating
around, the eye. The patient is prostrated, nauseated, and may even vomit,
while vision may be reduced to a bare perception of light. On examination
there is a dusky ciliary congestion, and the cornea appears steamy (due to
the corneal oedema collecting under the epithelium as minute blisters).
The congestion of the iris will make the anterior chamber more than
usually shallow, and the iris itself will be seen (albeit darkly through the
misty cornea) to be dull grey and patternless owing to the oedema; the
pupil is generally dilated, vertically oval, and fixed to light (Plate 5,
following p. 60). The ocular tension is of a stony hardness (Fig. 3.11).

haloes around lights

When these bouts of ocular hypertension are mild and transient, they
suffice only to cause a little oedema of the cornea without any pain or
congestion, as a result of which the patient sees coloured haloes around
lights—a *subacute glaucoma*. Such mild attacks do little, if any, damage to
the retinal elements, but they are danger signals, since they may well be

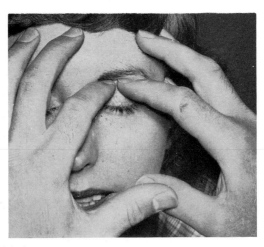

Fig. 3.11. Digital tonometry.

early cataract → windowed holes *wavy migraine*

followed by the dramatic onslaught of the acute attack; while to the old-hand they may simply serve as benevolent reminders that the pilocarpine drops are overdue. These glaucoma haloes may be mimicked by the diffusion of light-points when seen through an early cataract (but then the halo is fairly constant and uncoloured), and by the scintillating auras of migraine.

TREATMENT

Since the attack is precipitated by a pupil dilation, *Eserine* (1 per cent) or *Pilocarpine* (4 per cent) drops should be inserted every few minutes in an attempt to constrict the pupil and so disencumber the angle of the anterior chamber. *Acetazolamide* (Diamox), 250 mg intramuscularly (and thereafter t.d.s. by mouth) will assist by inhibiting aqueous production. Meanwhile the pain and photophobia can be allayed by analgesics, and eye-pad and heat.

If the eye is very hard, the cornea may be too waterlogged to permit much ingress of the pupil-constricting drops, and inhibition of aqueous production is of little benefit when there is already no room for more aqueous to enter; in this case a draught of *glycerol* (75 ml in water or lemon juice) may well be effective in dehydrating the eye by its osmotic effect in the blood. This can be achieved more surely, but more laboriously, by an intra-venous infusion of mannitol. Only when these measures fail is surgical decompression necessary, usually by the classical emergency

DIFFERENTIAL DIAGNOSIS

	Acute conjunctivitis	Acute iritis	Acute glaucoma
Pain	grittiness	moderate to severe	severe and radiating
Discharge	often purulent	slight reflex epiphora only	
Photophobia	mild	severe	moderate
Cornea	bright and clear	K.P.	epithelial oedema
Pupil	normal	consticted, fixed; later irregular from adhesions	dilated, oval, fixed
Iris	normal	muddy	greenish-grey
Tension	normal	normal (tender)	very hard (very tender)

festooned post synechiae! *haloe*

operation of a *Glaucoma Iridectomy* (in which a wide sector of the iris is excised).

Once the attack has been controlled, or the subacute 'haloes' correctly diagnosed, a régime of pilocarpine drops (1–2 per cent b.d.) is necessary to maintain a constricted pupil, and so prevent a further congestive attack until prophylactic surgery can be arranged (these drops are generally needed in both eyes, since the tendency is normally bilateral). The classical prophylactic operation is a Peripheral Iridectomy, making a small hole through the iris root, so as to allow free passage of aqueous between anterior and posterior chambers. However, if the attack has been prolonged, and the oedematous iris root has remained in contact with the peripheral cornea for too long, they may adhere; such 'peripheral anterior synechias' (which can be inspected through a 'gonioscopic lens') will then permanently impede the escape of aqueous, and the condition comes to resemble a 'simple glaucoma' (p. 52), and calls for excision also of a segment of sclera, to allow the aqueous to disperse into the subconjunctival lymphatics.

ACUTE KERATITIS

Keratitis may be exogenous or endogenous. The former is much more common, since the cornea is exposed throughout life to a succession of minor traumas, and the conjunctival sac is a favourite harbour for pathogenic bacteria; such an exogenous keratitis thus first involves the superficial corneal layers, and, since the epithelium has normally been disrupted, presents as a *corneal ulcer*. Endogenous keratities, due to systemic allergy or toxins, start deep in the cornea; they are an ill-assorted group, usually of obscure origin, but including one important clinical entity, due to congenital syphilis—*interstitial keratitis.*

Corneal ulcers

Generally of two main groups: (1) The small multiple *marginal ulcers* (Fig. 3.12), due to a severe conjunctival infection, usually with staphylococcus aureus, which transgresses the corneal margin; they are generally mild, clear away with routine antibiotic applications, and cause no ultimate impairment of vision. (2) The larger *central ulcer* (Fig. 3.13) which is usually single; this may be due to bacteria (particularly the pneumococcus) that has entered after an abrasion or alongside a corneal foreign body; more often nowadays it is the herpes simplex virus which provokes a

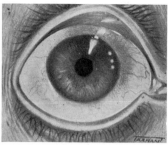

Fig. 3.12. Marginal corneal ulcers. Catarrhal ulcers, secondary to a conjunctival infection.

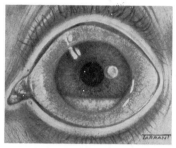

Fig. 3.13. Pneumococcal corneal ulcer with a typical hypopyon, the ulcer is spreading medially beneath an overhanging edge.

superficial but indolent 'dendritic ulcer' (Fig. 3.14), so-called because of its characteristic pattern. Such herpetic infections usually start as a stomatitis (often contracted by kissing), and a relapsing corneal infection follows, which is perpetuated by persistence of the virus in the mouth, and is commonly aggravated by the indiscriminate use of topical steroids which do deceptively allay the redness of the eye (just as morphia may deceptively ease an acute abdomen).

Central ulcers also occasionally arise when the cornea is dessicated or devitalized, as this area is farthest from the nutrient blood vessels at the corneo-scleral margins (e.g. following long-standing iritis, in keratites associated with skin diseases as acne rosacea, and in keratomalacia due to lack of vitamin A) and from over-exposure (e.g. where the lids cannot adequately protect the cornea, as in endocrine exophthalmos or facial palsy). Similar punctate erosions of the exposed area of the cornea can follow exposure to ultraviolet light as in 'arc-eye' from welding flashes or snow-blindness (milder exposure leads only to conjunctival congestion); these clear within a few days without residual damage.

SIGNS AND SYMPTOMS

These are essentially a composite of the signs and symptoms of the underlying conjunctivitis (irritation, conjunctival injection, discharge), augmented by those of the mild iritis (boring pain, ciliary injection, impaired vision) especially with the more infiltrating central ulcer; in the latter the seepage of toxins through the anterior chamber, may provoke an exudate of pus which gravitates as a hypopyon (Fig. 3.15). In addition the ulcer itself will be apparent as a cloudy opacity in the cornea; this can be confirmed to be an actual ulcer (and not just a scar from previous ulceration, in an eye which is injected for some incidental reason), by demonstrating that the overlying epithelium is deficient, since insertion of

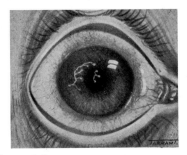

Fig. 3.14. Dendritic corneal ulcer.

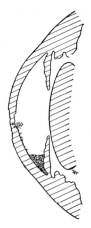

Fig. 3.15. Section of cornea with pneumococcal ulcer, showing hypopyon and purulent deposit on the posterior corneal surface.

a vital stain such as fluorescein into the conjunctival sac, will stain the exposed area bright green. The visual loss will be correspondingly great if the ulcer is large and central.

Only the most severe corneal ulcers progress to perforation, such as those due to infantile gonococcal conjunctivitis (ophthalmia neonatorum) or the central ulcer caused by the rare but devastating contaminant of eyedrops—pseudomonas aeruginosa. Even then the iris generally falls forward to plug the hole, and leaving an anterior synechia up to the base of the scar (Plate 13, following p. 60), when the inflammation subsides.

TREATMENT

This correspondingly entails a combination of the treatment for the underlying conjunctival infection (*antibiotic* drops, etc.) plus that for the secondary iritis (*atropine, heat, pad*, but not corticosteroids, which delay epithelial regeneration). In the case of dendritic ulcers, the specific anti-viral drops of *idoxuridene* are effective if given frequently (every hour) in the early stages; and steroid drops have an especial danger in promoting an extension of the ulcer.

Various further measures may be required if, as is all too frequent, the ulcer is indolent. *Carbolization* (painting the corneal surface with pure carbolic acid, after instilling anaesthetic drops) often expedites recovery. A *Tarsorrhaphy* (suturing the lids together) may be required to give added protection if the corneal sensation is lowered ('neurotrophic keratitis'), as in the fairly common herpes zoster of the ophthalmic division of the trigeminal nerve, or where the lids cannot cover the eye as after a facial palsy ('neuroparalytic keratitis'), or because of a severe exophthalmos.

Interstitial keratitis

This is one of the late stigmas of congenital syphilis (although milder forms very occasionally occur in acquired syphilis, tuberculosis, etc.); it develops about puberty, and one eye follows its fellow a few months later. Both corneas become very oedematous, and subsequently pink with the ingrowth of new blood vessels from the adjacent sclera (Fig. 3.16); after some months of pain and virtual blindness, the periphery of the cornea begins to clear, leaving only a diffuse cloudiness in the central area, so that the majority of cases regain enough vision to read ordinary print. The actual cause is probably an anaphylactic reaction to the spirochaetal endotoxin, and the treatment is thus palliative until the disease has run its

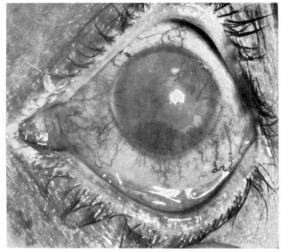

Fig. 3.16. Interstitial keratitis. Generalized haze with ingrowth of pallisade of deep corneal blood-vessels. (Cook.)

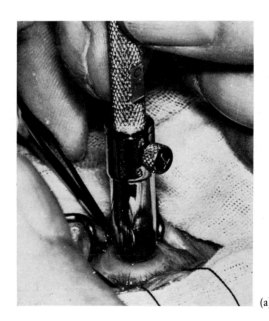

(a)

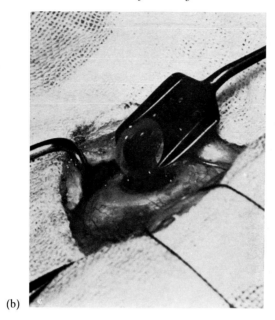

(b)

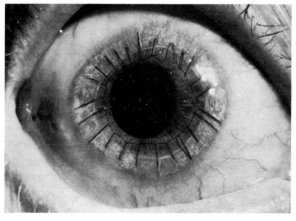

(c)

Fig. 3.17 *opposite and above.* Corneal graft. (*a*) Trephining the recipient cornea.
(*b*) Sliding the donor corneal disc into place. (*c*) Graft sutured in position.

course, entailing drops of *corticosteroid* (which can reduce the intensity of the oedema and vascularization, and therewith the ultimate scarring) and *atropine* (an intense iritis is a normal, if concealed accompaniment). Anti-syphilitic therapy is usually given, in the hope that it may prevent a subsequent gummatous or nervous lesion.

When the attack is over, the resulting corneal scars ('nebulae' if faint, or 'leucomata' if dense) are especially amenable for replacement by grafts from the cornea of a healthy cadaver eye. (Fig. 3.17). These grafts, usually discs of the full corneal thickness, about 7 mm in diameter, are sewn into the place of an identically sized disc of damaged cornea. They normally remain clear, since (unlike homografts of other tissues) the cornea is avascular and excites little antigenic reaction, and even if they do become opaque, the 'keratoplasty' can always be repeated. Such grafts may be justified for therepeutic as well as optical reasons, replacing corneas which are devitalized (as after indolent herpes simplex infections) or eroded (and liable to perforate).

Cadaver eyes are in short supply, as their cornea becomes unsuitable for grafting within a few days unless it is 'deep-frozen'; but eye-banks are now established in most major cities. In England patients may bequeath their eyes for grafting, and the eyes can then be taken without obtaining the consent of their executors, providing the surviving spouse or relatives do not object.

Scleritis, or 'episcleritis'

Since the vascular superficial laminae of the sclera are principally involved, this is one further cause of painful red eye. It arises generally as a form of collagen degeneration, essentially comparable to rheumatic nodules elsewhere in the body.

The eye becomes red, but this congestion is localized and indurated (unlike that of a generalized conjunctivitis) (Plate 6, following p. 60), and the patient experiences a constant dull ache, rather than a 'grittiness' on movements of the upper lid; in the more severe cases there are signs of an underlying iritis. The disease lasts a few weeks, with a tendency to relapses; but the discomfort can be allayed by topical steroids (systemically, if necessary) and these can be used symptomatically until the bout passes. Oral salicylates and topical heat will also relieve the discomfort.

CHAPTER 4
GRADUAL LOSS OF SIGHT IN
QUIET EYES

Blindness in England is caused, in the main, by three diseases:—Cataract (23 per cent), Glaucoma (13 per cent) and Senile degeneration of the macula (27 per cent). In nearly all cases these develop insidiously in the elderly; but whereas cataract can be remedied, glaucoma can only be arrested, and retinal degenerations ruthlessly progress.

CATARACT

The lens is avascular, and its cells (apart from the anterior epithelium) lose their nuclei and therefore cannot divide; their only function is to remain transparent, and their only response to any insult—developmental mishap, inflammation, disordered metabolism, trauma or radiation—is to become opaque, so forming a 'cataract'. However, the large majority of cataracts represent a simple senile change, corresponding to the degeneration of other epidermal derivatives such as the whitening of the hair, and some degree of lens opacity is found in the majority of patients over 60.

SIGNS AND SYMPTOMS

The cardinal symptom is a gradual failure of sight, and the cardinal sign is a white opacity within the pupil (Fig. 4.1). In its early stages the cataract may be barely visible on direct illumination, but presents ophthalmoscopically as a silhouette against the red fundus reflex, often localized to the lens nucleus, or else as flakes, dots or sector-shaped opacities within the lens periphery (Fig. 4.2).

TREATMENT

Opacification of the lens is irreversible, since the protein becomes denatured as in a hard-boiled egg; so the only treatment of such an opacity is to remove it by operation. This can be performed at any age or any stage in its development, and is normally advised whenever the cataract becomes a

47

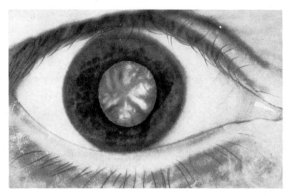

Fig. 4.1. Mature cataract: a white opacity within the pupil.

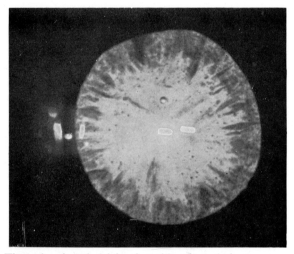

Fig. 4.2. The wedge-shaped peripheral opacities of a cortical cataract, presenting on ophthalmoscopy as silhouettes against the red fundus reflex.

sufficient impediment to the patient's normal activities—generally when it interferes with reading (this corresponds roughly to the time when the vision in the better eye is reduced to 6/18), and then the cataract is removed from the worse eye, if (as is usual) both are affected. Beneath the age of 35 removal of the whole lens nearly always leads to a damaging escape of vitreous, but as these youthful lenses have no hardened nucleus, it will suffice to tear open the anterior lens capsule with a needle (cf. Fig. 4.6), so that the aqueous can mix freely with the opaque soft lens matter, which will gradually be washed away into the blood stream; such 'need-lings' may need to be repeated several times before all the opaque lens matter disperses, and it is often better simply to aspirate this through a wide-bore needle. However over the age of 35 the nucleus of the lens becomes increasingly hard, and must be lifted out through an incision in the eyeball along its corneo-scleral margin. The standard form of this operation involves the removal of the entire lens—and 'intra-capsular extraction'—grasping its tenuous capsule with forceps (Fig. 4.3) or, more simply and securely, by adhering the lens periphery to a freezing 'cryo-probe'. The whole lens is then gently lifted out of the eye (Fig. 4.4). In the older method—and 'extra-capsular extraction'—the capsule is simply torn open (as in the operation of 'needling') and the hard lens nucleus squeezed out through the incision (Fig. 4.5). This extra-capsular method, although technically easier, has the disadvantage that the capsule which has been left behind will need to be punctured several weeks later (a 'capsulotomy' Fig. 4.6), before the light rays can have unimpeded access to the retina.

After cataract extraction, thick convex spectacle-lenses are needed to replace the convex 'crystalline lens' that has been removed from within the eye, and then full vision can usually be restored. The retinal image, as seen

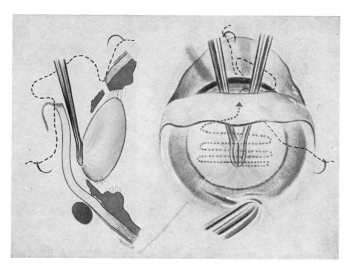

Fig. 4.3. Cataract extraction. The intracapsular technique, grasping the thin capsule with forceps, gradually dislocating it by side-to-side movements, and then somersaulting the entire lens out through the limbal incision. Counter-pressure is applied by a blunt hook at the lower corneal margin.

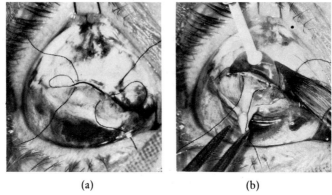

(a)　　　　　　　　　　　　　　　(b)

Fig. 4.4. Cryo-extraction of cataract. (*a*) A flap of conjunctiva has been turned back, the limbus incised, and sutures inserted. (*b*) The cataract is pulled out, adhering to the freezing-probe.

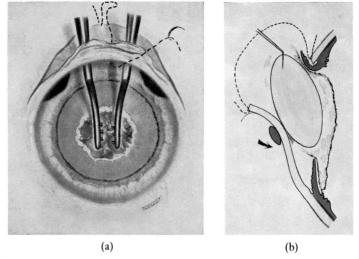

(a)　　　　　　　　　　　　　　　(b)

Fig. 4.5. Cataract extraction. Extracapsular technique (*a*) preliminary avulsion of central part of the anterior lens capsule, and (*b*) expression of the lens nucleus through this gap in the capsule and out through the limbal incision, easing it away with a sharp hook as it emergies.

through the convex spectacle lens in front of (instead of within) the eyeball, is then a third larger in size; and, if the fellow eye has fairly good vision the two images cannot be fused, so that the patient sees double if both eyes are wearing their proper spectacle correction. This often perplexes the patient who finds the optical problem difficult to comprehend; and, although contact lenses may reduce the image-size of the aphakic eye near enough to permit fusion, senile patients cannot usually cope with these, and it may be necessary to black-out the spectacle lens of the unoperated eye. In addition to this problem of the monocular aphakic, the new world, as seen through cataract spectacles, is often daunting, when the objects they see, already too large and with their straight edges curved,

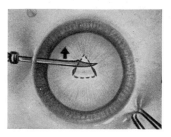

Fig. 4.6. Capsulotomy. Division of the thickened posterior capsule or 'after-cataract' with a needle-knife; here a tongue-shaped flap is being cut, which will fall downwards with gravity and leave a clear central gap in the capsular remnant.

squirm about with every eye-movement or pop in and out of the peripheral blind areas with the insolence of a jack-in-the-box; and months of patience and perseverance are usually needed before the frailer psyches can cope with this formidable new visual world.

Congenital cataracts

These vary in size from an entirely opaque lens to the occasional dots that can be seen in most normal lenses and cause no visual impediment. Some are hereditary; others are specifically attributable to maternal disease, thus cataract is an almost invariable sequel to rubella when this is contracted within the first eight weeks of pregnancy, and a 'lamellar cataract' (shaped like a plate in the posterior lens cortex, with its thickened rim generally just concealed by the pupil margin—Fig. 4.7) is often the result of a lowered blood calcium just before or after birth.

Binocular congenital cataracts should be cleared within a few months of birth, if they are dense enough to prevent the development of macular fixation; otherwise, or if uniocular, their removal can be deferred for a few years, until detailed assessment and the operation are easier.

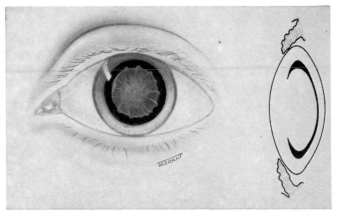

Fig. 4.7. Lamellar cataract. The position of this plate-shaped opacity within the lens is shown in the diagram alongside.

Secondary cataracts

Cataracts may be secondary to *trauma* (concussion, or an actual rupture of the lens capsule from a perforating wound), *intra-ocular inflammation* (by impeding its metabolism, or by frank toxins from a protracted irido-cyclitis), *endocrine upset* (adolescent diabetics may be blinded by a sudden snowflake-like deposit throughout the lens cortex, although this has become rare since the widespread use of insulin, and elderly diabetics are more prone to develop an ordinary senile cataract; cataracts may also form in aparathyroidea, due to lowered blood calcium-, inborn *metabolic* defect (as galactosaemia and homocystinuria), *radiation* (high voltage X-rays and infra-red rays).

SIMPLE GLAUCOMA

When the intra-ocular pressure is raised very gradually over many months, all the acute manifestations of a congestive glaucomatous attack are lacking, since the eye remains white and painless; but the damage to the retina and optic nerve fibres, which in the acute attack is dramatic, is here so insidious that it is easily overlooked by the patient (or by the untrained practitioner) until much of the sight is irretrievably lost.

The aetiology of simple glaucoma is obscure, since the anterior chamber is of normal depth and there is no overt obstruction to the drainage angle. It is probably, in the main, a senile sclerotic process of the smaller intra-ocular vessels, and secondarily of the ocular tissues; in the anterior segment of the eye this sclerosis obstructs the aqueous outflow, and so elevates intra-ocular pressure, while posteriorly it leads to ischaemic atrophy of the fibres in the optic nerve-head which causes both the atrophic cupping of the disc and restriction of the visual fields. The elevated pressure thus damages the sight only indirectly, by aggraving the ischaemic changes of the posterior segment.

SIGNS AND SYMPTOMS

1. *The intra-ocular pressure is raised*, although the eyeball is not so hard as in an attack of glaucoma. The pressure, which can be crudely assessed by fluctuating the down-turned eyeball with the forefingers, can be measured more exactly by a simple tonometer which records the degree a plunger will impress the (anaesthetized) cornea (Fig. 4.9); or one which is attached to the corneal microscope and records the weight required to flatten a standard area of the corneal dome.

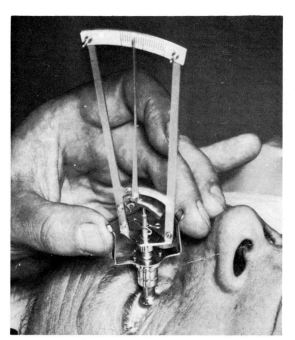

Fig. 4.8. Tonometry, with Schiötz tonometer.

2. *The vision is gradually destroyed.* This loss starts as a blind patch—a 'scotoma', which soon forms an upward or downward extension of the normal blind-spot, and reaches to join an indentation of the peripheral field in the upper or lower nasal quadrants (Fig. 4.9); and it progresses till only a small patch of the central vision remains, although within this surviving island the acuity is barely affected. Finally, the eye becomes quite blind.

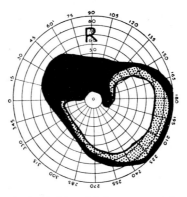

Fig. 4.9. The field-loss in simple (chronic) glaucoma: peripheral encroachment in the upper nasal sector has become confluent with the 'arcuate' scotoma which extends upwards from the normal blind-spot. (The blacked-out area represents that part of the normal visual field which has been totally lost, and within this is a stippled area where vision is present but impaired.)

3. *The optic disc is cupped,* and at the same time becomes white and 'atrophic'. This must be differentiated from physiological cupping, which is simply an exaggeration of the central pit, does not reach the disc margin, and is not atrophic (Plate 7a and b, following p. 60).

TREATMENT

As for acute bouts of closed-angle glaucoma, treatment consists essentially in attempting to control the tension with miotic drops (as pilocarpine up to 4 per cent g.d.s.) and Diamox tablets, and where this fails—as evidenced by a persistently raised pressure or a continued encroachment of the visual fields on charting every few months—a surgical decompression of the eye. But whereas the acute glaucoma is due to an overt mechanical block which (after initial medical control) needs surgical rectification, the treatment of simple glaucoma is essentially medical, and surgery to create new exit passage for the aqueous is only a last resort.

Diamox is less valuable here than in acute glaucoma, but should supplement the miotics in cases with a high tension which are less suitable for surgery; and neutral adrenalin drops will also reduce aqueous secretion (especially helpful when the small pupil is an embarrassment, as in the presence of central lens opacities).

The standard operation is the sclerectomy, in which a small strip of sclera at the upper corneal margin is removed (as well as a knuckle of the underlying iris root), so the the aqueous under pressure can filter out through the hole and disperse into the subconjunctival lymphatics; traditionally this piece of sclera is excised by a circular 'trephine' (Fig. 4.10), but nowadays a knife and scissors are usually preferred (Fig. 4.11) with cautery to the scleral lip, to help it to stay open. As an alternative, a wick of iris tissue may be drawn out through the corneo-scleral incision, to produce there a spongy filtering scar—an 'iridencleisis'. Sometimes these drainage operations need repetition, or need to be supplemented by further miotic drops; and even then the degenerative process may continue, albeit retarded, to destroy the sight.

Congenital glaucoma

Glaucoma may also result from maldevelopment at the drainage-angle of

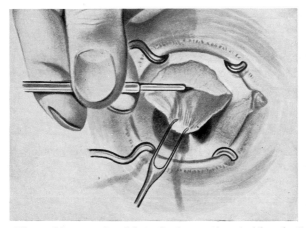

Fig. 4.10. The trephine operation. After reflecting a conjunctival flap, the disc of corneo-sclera is excised by rotating the trephine between the fingers.

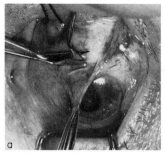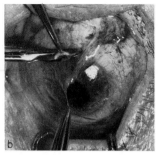

Fig. 4.11. Sclerectomy. (*a*) After the limbal incision, a knuckle of iris is removed. (*b*) The strip of sclera is excised.

the anterior chamber. The soft infantile sclera distends under the increased intra-ocular pressure, so that these swollen eyes look ox-like and the condition is thus called *Buphthalmos* (Fig. 4.12). The essential treatment is to open-up, at an early stage, the occluded angle of the anterior chamber by the sweep of a 'goniotomy' knife (under direct vision through a gonioscopic lens); the eye must be examined regularly under anaesthetic, with further goniotomies if the hypertension persists.

DEGENERATION OF THE RETINA AND CHOROID

A miscellany of degenerative fundus changes, beyond the range of treatment, are a common cause of gradual visual loss in old age; they are ascribed to a genetic lowering of vitality of the neural or vascular elements of the choroid and retina, and generally labelled 'dystrophies' or 'abiotrophies'. They are usually localized to the macular area.

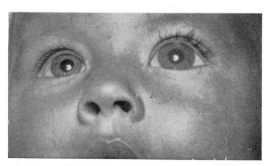

Fig. 4.12. Buphthalmos. The left eyeball is distended, and its cornea rendered hazy with oedema.

Senile macular degeneration presents clinically with an insidious bilateral *central scotoma*; and the corresponding area of macula becomes mottled with pigment (Fig. 4.13), a change that is easily overlooked in the earliest stages, but in some cases the whole area may become swollen with exudate or spattered with blood and haemorrhagic residues. Such patients may be assisted by certain optical devices (as telescopic spectacles), but the involuting mind adapts tardily, and a simple hand-magnifying-lens often serves them best. These macular degenerations may occur in young adults

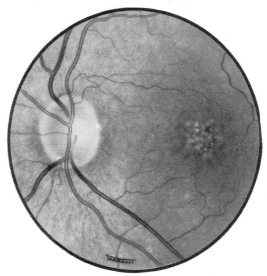

Fig. 4.13. Senile macular degeneration.

or even infancy, having then a more obvious hereditary-familial basis, being proportionately more rapid, and, in the youngest groups such as Tay-Sachs disease, being accompanied by degenerative changes in other tissues that are usually fatal. Similar pigmentary degenerative changes at the macula may be the legacy of prolonged dosage with toxic drugs, such as chloroquine.

Retinitis pigmentosa is the commonest of the dystrophies that cause a loss of the *peripheral* vision; it sometimes presents with a night-blindness, since the retinal periphery is largely responsible for night-vision. The fundus shows a striking scattering of black pigment, in patterns resembling bone-corpuscles, at first involving the equatorial region but finally over all but the posterior pole (Fig. 4.14). Degeneration of the retinal elements starts in adolescence, progresses remorselessly, and is attested by an increasing retinal pigmentation and a deepening pallor of the optic disc as the ganglion cells die. Retinitis pigmentosa is more strictly genetically determined, occurring in various syndromes (e.g. along with polydactyly, obesity etc. in 'Lawrence-Moon-Biedl syndrome'), and carriers of the gene may show depression of the electrical retinal responses before the retinal pigmentation becomes apparent.

In very exceptional cases, the progress of a SMD may be delayed by

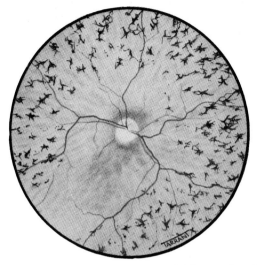

Fig. 4.14. Retinitis pigmentosa. The 'bone-corpuscle' pigment-deposits are restricted to the retinal periphery.

laser coagulation of leaking paramacular vessels. But no treatment will delay that of retinitis pigmentosa; however its irregular course has fostered many panaceas, with no clinical justification.

Atrophy of the choroido-retina is also a classical sequel to foci of **choroiditis**; and the exposed white sclera, together with occasional patches where the retinal pigment-epithelium has proliferated, may give an appearance resembling the foregoing primary retinal degenerations, except that the areas involved are usually irregular and, if bilateral, rarely symmetrical (Plate 8, following p. 60). The visual loss is also stationary and dates from a bout (often unremembered) of impaired vision due to the vitreous exudation during the acute attack. The aetiology of acute choroiditis, as with iritis, is generally unknown, although serological tests attribute a fair proportion to toxoplasmosis; but in the treatment, since there is no pain or photophobia, heat and pad are unnecessary, and atropine has little influence on its evolution; topical corticosteroids barely penetrate to the posterior segment of the eye, so prednisolone (5–15 mg t.d.s.) is usually prescribed until the acute attack subsides.

A similar choroido-retinal atrophy occurs in **high myopia** (or 'progressive myopia'), when it is restricted to the area of the macula and around the optic disc. There is proportionate loss of central vision, which is often sudden if small retinal tears or haemorrhages appear.

Both acute choroiditis and high myopia are characterized by opacities in the vitreous, caused respectively by inflammatory exudate and by degenerative changes in the gel as the eyeball elongates; and when these opacities are sufficiently dense, or so placed that they cast discrete shadows on the retina, they become visible to the patient, and are seen to float with each movement of the eye. Minor 'floaters' occur in healthy eyes as wisps and dots, which are barely visible except against an even light background; they have no pathological significance, and are aptly known as *muscae volitantes* (flitting flies).

CHAPTER 5
SUDDEN LOSS OF SIGHT IN QUIET EYES

The gradual extinction of sight in one eye may well be overlooked by the incurious or obtuse patient, and the presence of a blind eye is then suddenly discovered when the seeing eye happens to be occluded; but a sudden loss of sight rarely passes unnoticed, however painless. This is normally the result of a vascular mishap—either blockage of the end-arteries or 'end-veins' of the retina, or a copious intra-ocular haemorrhage; or else only a part of the visual field may be lost, following a retinal detachment or a thrombosis within the optic tracts or radiations—including the relatively common homonymous hemianopia that follows a thrombosis of the posterior cerebral vessels. Since the former group devolve in the main from retinal arterio-sclerosis and the related retinopathies, these may first be briefly considered, although to some extent they fall more within the ambit of general medicine.

RETINAL ARTERIOSCLEROSIS

The following pathological changes in the retinal arteries can be discerned (Fig. 5.1):

1. **Spasm**—often intermittent and localized. The blood columns then appear narrowed (the vessel walls themselves are normally invisible); and the retina may appear opalescent from oedema (the retina itself is also normally invisible, and the fundus background is formed by the blood in choroidal vessels with their associated pigment, faintly screened by the single layer of the retinal pigmentepithelium).

2. **Sclerosis**—a thickening of the arterial walls which gives the heart an added load, although if a raised systolic pressure can be maintained, retinal function is unimpaired. This is shown ophthalmoscopically by the vessel walls themselves becoming opaque, with at first a bright surface reflex ('copper-wire arteries'), which may ultimately conceal the underlying blood-column ('silver-wire arteries'); at the same time the hardened arteries press on the veins at their crossings, interrupting, and later deflecting the venous column.

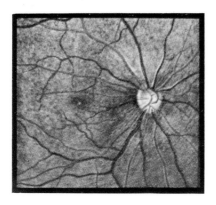

PLATE I (*see page 2*).
The negroid fundus. (Perkins and Hansell, *Diseases of the Eye.*)

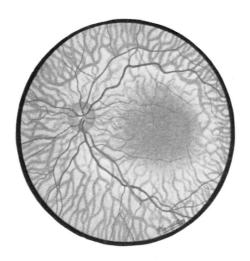

PLATE 2 (*see page 2*).
The albinoid fundus. (Hamblin.)

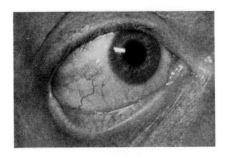

PLATE 3 (*see page 18*).
Pinguecula.

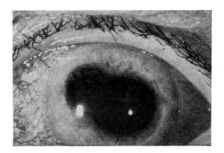

PLATE 4 (*see page 34*).
Acute iritis, with ciliary injection and festooned pupil due to the posterior synechias which had formed before atropine was instilled.

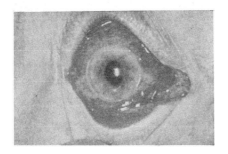

PLATE 5 (*see page 38*).
Acute glaucoma, with ciliary injection, oval, semi-dilated pupil and corneal haze.

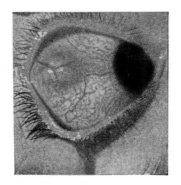

PLATE 6 (*see page 46*).
Episcleritis. (Gifford's *Textbook of Ophthalmology*.)

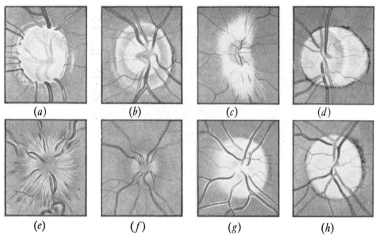

(a)   (b)   (c)   (d)

(e)   (f)   (g)   (h)

PLATE 7 (*see pages 6, 54, 78, 89, 91*).

(*a*) Glaucomatous cupping of the optic disc.

(*b*) Physiological cupping of the optic disc.

(*c*) Opaque nerve fibres spreading onto the adjacent retina.

(*d*) The optic disc in myopia—enlarged by a crescent of exposed sclera.

(*e*) Papilloedema.

(*f*) The optic disc in high hypermetropia ('pseudo-papilloedema').

(*g*) Post-neuritic ('secondary') optic atrophy.

(*h*) Simple ('primary') optic atrophy.

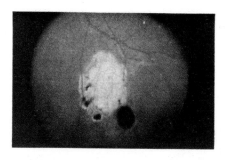

PLATE 8 (*see page 58*).
Scarring from focus of choroiditis.

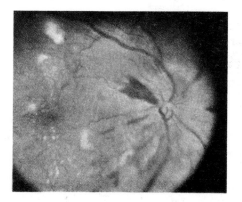

Plate 9 (*see page 61*).
Retinopathy in malignant hypertension. Fundus photograph showing gross oedema of optic disc and adjacent retina, with superficial haemorrhages and scattered 'cotton-wool exudates'.

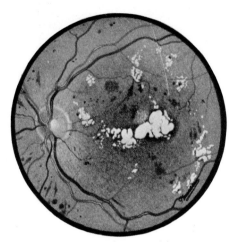

PLATE 10 (*see page 62*).
Diabetic retinopathy, with small deep haemorrhages and hard
exudates.

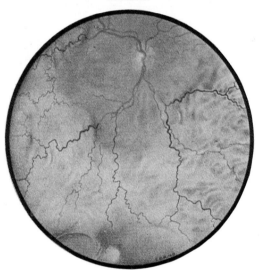

PLATE 11 (*see page 67*).
Retinal detachment.

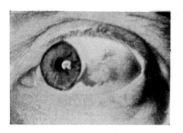

PLATE 12 (*see page 70*).
Subconjunctival haemorrhage.

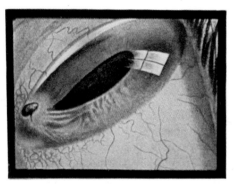

PLATE 13 (*see pages 43, 73*).
Perforating corneal wound near the lower corneal margin, this
has become plugged by 'prolapsed' iris, which forms a black
knuckle externally. (Hamblin.)

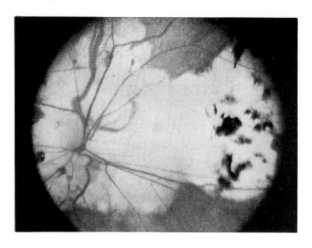

PLATE 14 (*see page 78*).

Chorio-retinal atrophy in high myopia. The usual temporal crescent has extended all the way around the disc, and this ring of exposed sclera has become confluent with that at the macular area.

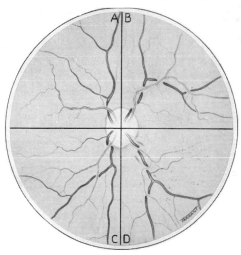

Fig. 5.1. Retinal arteriosclerosis. The four quadrants illustrate the sequence of vascular changes, with increasing evidence of pressure at the arterio-venous crossings, increasing attenuation and irregularity of the arteries, and finally scattered haemorrhages and exudates in the retina.

3. **Constriction** of the blood column, when intimal proliferation encroaches on the lumen.

4. **Retinopathy**—with *haemorrhages*, which being superficial are flame-shaped (since they spread tangentially among the fibres of the inner layer of the retina, as these converge towards the optic disc), and also some small *hard exudates*. These various deposits may cause little visual impairment and constantly clear away, to be replaced by haemorrhages and exudates elsewhere.

Malignant hypertension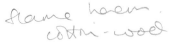

Malignant hypertension differs essentially from the foregoing fundus picture of benign hypertension in showing a generalized arterial spasm, leading to gross retinal oedema, which may spread onto the disc (as papilloedema), along with areas of retinal necrosis ('cotton-wool patches') (Plate 9, following p. 60).

Renal retinopathy

A hypertensive-arteriosclerotic retinopathy may be augmented when the toxic metabolites due to reduced kidney function further damage the retinal arterial walls, rendering them more permeable; so that oedema, then exudates, and finally haemorrhages appear. These latter are all variable in amount and constantly changing; the exudates characteristically form a fan-shaped pattern around the macula, and may entirely disappear before death (which usually follows within a year if untreated (Fig. 5.2).

macular – fan.

Diabetic retinopathy   *dot + blot. haem (deep)*
hard exudate

10–20 years after the onset of diabetes, some retinopathy is usually evident; the majority of cases are thus middle-aged, so that the signs of diabetic retinopathy are often complicated by the coincident signs of retinal arteriosclerosis. The primary lesion is a multitude of 'micro-aneurysms'; these are minute varicosities, just visible ophthalmoscopically, which later tend to leak and form haemorrhages, small and dark because they are deep within the retinal substance—producing the characteristic 'dot and blot' appearance (Plate 10, following p. 60). The exudates, which appear some years later, are also small, with 'hard' irregular edges, like pieces of cheese. These changes become gradually more profuse as the sight is destroyed, and blindness is often precipitated by a massive haemorrhage into the vitreous. In these earlier stages, no treatment will influence the progress of the retinopathy, but when the retinal vessels start

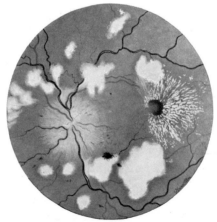

Fig. 5.2. Renal retinopathy, with haemorrhages, 'cotton wool exudates' and linear 'hard exudates' radiating like a fan around the macula.

to proliferate on the disc, or retinal oedema starts to endanger the central vision, obliteration of the new or leaking vessels (or else of the vascular bed at the retinal periphery) may sometimes be justified by a laser or photo-coagulator beam.

OCCLUSION OF THE CENTRAL RETINAL ARTERY

The central retinal artery may be blocked by spasm, by degenerative changes within its wall, or by an embolus; arterial occlusion is thus most common in the elderly arteriosclerotic, but may occur in the young adult with cardiovascular disease.

Sudden blindness is here associated with a classical fundus picture (Fig. 5.3), the arteries becoming transformed into narrow threads, and the whole fundus appearing milky white as the oedematous retina loses its trasparency; a day or two later a 'cherry-red spot' appears at the macula (where the retina is thin and the red choroid shows through, in contrast to the adjacent pallor), and by the time the retinal oedema has faded an optic atrophy is generally apparent.

When occlusion of the artery or its branches is simply due to spasm, this may relax within an hour or two, and vision return; otherwise blindness is complete, although an aberrant vascular supply to a patch of retina may occasionally salvage an island of sight. Antispasmotics are usually

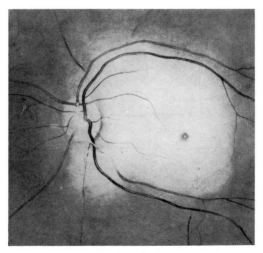

Fig. **5.3**. Occlusion of the central retinal artery.

administered, but with little prospect of success if the block has persisted more than a few hours.

When only a branch of the central artery is occluded, only the corresponding sector of retina is affected, leaving an appropriate scotoma. Transient retinal arterial occlusions are sometimes associated with contralateral hemipareses, due to recurrent emboli from atheroma in the common carotid arteries (which may lead to a massive cerebral vascular accident, if left untreated). Occlusion of the central retinal artery (or, less often, of the vein) is also a common sequel in the elderly to Giant-cell arteritis involving the arterioles around the optic disc. This diagnosis should always be suspected, and will often be confirmed by finding a raised E.S.R. Treatment with systemic steroids may then reduce the secondary oedema of the optic nerve head, and prevent a similar catastrophe in the fellow-eye.

OCCLUSION OF THE CENTRAL RETINAL VEIN

The central retinal vein is generally occluded by pressure of its escort artery at the optic disc, especially in the presence of venous congestion; occasionally occlusion is due to a toxic endophlebitis. Thus, like arterial occlusion, it is more common in the elderly arteriosclerotic, but again may arise in younger adults (usually women).

Here the loss of sight is a little less abrupt and less complete; and there is an equally arresting, but contrasting, fundus picture, with haemorrhages scattered riotously over the whole retina, irregular and superficial like bundles of straw alongside the retinal veins, which are themselves tortuous and very engorged. After a few weeks the haemorrhages gradually clear, and little trace of the initial onslaught ultimately remains, apart from the occasional but pathognomonic formation of new anastomotic vessels on the disc; however, the sight may show scant improvement. Treatment is of no avail, but as retinal venous thrombosis is more common in eyes prone to simple glaucoma, the latter must be excluded in the fellow eye.

The tranquil course of resolution is interrupted after about three months in nearly 20 per cent of cases by an acute secondary glaucoma, which expunges the little sight that remains. This follows obstructions of the drainage angle by new vessels which form on the iris root owing to the secondary retinal hypoxia, and no treatment is merited except for the symptomatic relief of pain (e.g. by retrobulbar injection of alcohol).

As often as not venous occlusion (with a secondary thrombosis) is limited to one of the four principal trunks (Fig. 5.4), with the obstruction

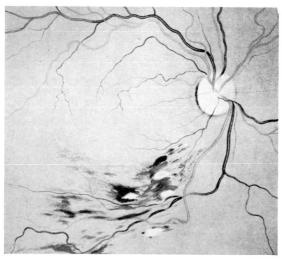

Fig. 5.4. Occlusion of the lower temporal branch of the central retinal vein.

visibly beginning at an arterio-venous crossing, and the damage will then be confined to the appropriate sector, the macula being involved if either the upper temporal or lower temporal veins are affected; but here the recovery of sight is usual, and there is no risk of a subsequent glaucoma.

VITREOUS HAEMORRHAGE

Retinal haemorrhages are seen to be a major component of the various retinopathies; they similarly develop in many blood diseases wherein haemorrhages are especially liable (anaemia, purpura, etc.), and particularly in an idiopathic disease of young adult males attributed to periphlebitis(?tuberculous) and named 'Eales' Disease'. When severe, they errupt into the vitreous cavity (a particular feature of Eales' disease, in which vitreous haemorrhages occur every few months over a period of several years); but sometimes they are restrained behind the hyaloid membrane that bounds the vitreous, and then appear as a characteristic **pre-retinal** or **subhyaloid** haemorrhage—forming an even film, with an outline which is circular, but which may develop a flattened upper margin as the corpuscles gravitate downwards (Fig. 5.5). Subhyaloid haemorrhages often accompany subarachnoid haemorrhage or subdural haematoma's, especially in early childhood. Vitreous haemorrhages clear very slowly;

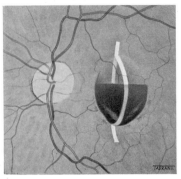

Fig. 5.5. Pre-retinal ('sub-hyaloid') haemorrhage, with its upper fluid level, contained between the posterior surface of the vitreous and the inner surface of the retina (these two surfaces are here illuminated by the vertical beam of light from a 'slit-lamp', which is coming in obliquely from the right-hand side).

only when they are extensive or often repeated are they liable to become organized, leaving the eye partially or completely blind. In such a case, surgical evacuation, with a complex 'vitrectomy' machine, is occasionally justified.

RETINAL DETACHMENT

In embryology the retina is formed by the invagination of an optic vesicle, its outer layer persisting as the single-celled layer of 'pigment epithelium', and its inner layer proliferating to form the rods, cones and the various cell-relays. The cavity of the optic vesicle persists as a potential space between these layers; and, if the inner layer should rupture, vitreous can seep in through the hole and open up this space, by displacing the visual layer of the retina forwards, as a 'retinal detachment'. Such ruptures generally occur in degenerate patches at the retinal periphery, which tend to adhere to the overlying vitreous, and which are most commonly found in the attenuated retina of an elongated myopic eye (p. 78); such a tear is usually initiated by trauma, which need be no more that a slight shaking if the retina is sufficiently degenerate.

SIGNS AND SYMPTOMS

The rods and cones over the detached area are thus separated from their choroidal blood supply and will ultimately die, so that to the patient is

flashes,
opacities

seems as if a curtain was descending (or ascending, if the detachment started above—corresponding to the lower visual field); and central vision is abruptly lost when the detachment spreads across the macular area. The antecedent retinal tear is often signalled by sudden flashes and floating opacities before the vision; and this warning signal should call for a careful inspection of the retinal periphery (under full mydriasis), as such tears can readily be sealed by coagulation if the retina is still in place. But if the retina has already detached, major surgery is needed, which may be unsuccessful, and always leaves some visual impairment. As retinal degeneration is usually bilateral, the fellow-eye must also be carefully checked.

Ophthalmoscopically the detached retina becomes apparent as an opalescent sheet 'ballooning' well forwards into the vitreous, and the initiating tear is usually visible, with the brilliant red choroid shining through it (Plate 11, following p. 60).

TREATMENT

If untended, the detachment normally becomes complete, and the eye blind. In about three-quarters of the cases the detachment can be arrested by sealing the retina back to choroid all around the hole, so blocking any

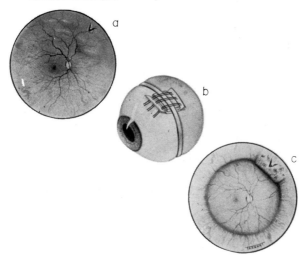

Fig. 5.6. Repair of retinal detachment. (*a*) Pre-operative fundus view, showing upper nasal U-shaped tear. (*b*) Encircling strap sutured in place (with plomb over site of tear). (*c*) Post-operative fundus view.

further seepage of vitreous fluid between the layers. This is achieved by invaginating the sclera and choroid towards the detached retina in the region of the retinal hole, and then the choroid and retina are made to adhere by the coagulating effect of a diathermy or freezing probe placed at appropriate sites on the overlying sclera (Fig. 5.6). Such coagulation can also be attained by an intense light-beam directed through the pupil ('photocoagulation'), and this simple procedure alone may suffice if the retina and choroid are already virtually in contact. Even in successful cases, a re-detachment may be initiated by some mild trauma to the head or by a physical effort such as stooping, especially in the myopic cases where the retina is already thin and degenerate; bed-rest is thus advised after the operation (and also pre-operatively to prevent any interim extension of the detached area).

Secondary retinal detachments

These are occasionally caused by a massive exudate between the two layers (as in the toxaemia of pregnancy) or a rapidly progressive neoplasm of the retina or choroid.

The two common primary malignant tumours of the eye are the **malignant melanoma** of the choroid, and a **retinoblastoma** of the

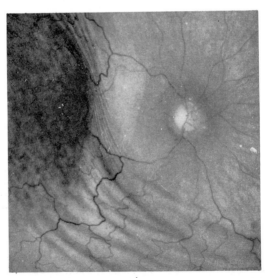

Fig. 5.7. Malignant melanoma, as seen on ophthalmoscopy, with the dark choroidal mass above, and a secondary fluid detachment below.

retina. Both progress until they fill the eyeball, often presenting when they obstruct the drainage angle and induce glaucoma; a third stage is that of local extra-ocular spread, and a fourth of distant metastases—the melanoma generally reaching the liver, and the retinoblastoma travelling up the optic nerve into the brain. The clinical picture of these tumours is otherwise very contrasting; the melanoma is uniocular, generally presenting in the middle-aged, as a dark oval mass, often concealed beneath a secondary retinal detachment (differentiation from a primary detachment is thus imperative but often difficult) (Fig. 5.7); while the retinoblastoma (Fig. 5.8) presents in early infancy as a white mass behind the pupil, to be differentiated from the residues of intra-uterine endophthalmitis, or a 'retrolental fibroplasia' (a maldevelopment largely due to administration of excessive oxygen to premature babies).

Eyes containing a large melanoma or retinoblastoma should be enucleated forthwith.* If the tumours are small, X-radiation, coagulation, or local excision may be safe; retinoblastomata are, however, often bilateral (and also familial), and the second eye must be carefully checked, lest a retinoblastoma has developed there also, requiring urgent treatment.

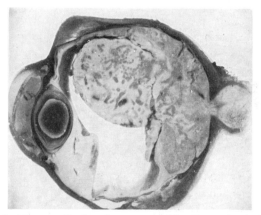

Fig. 5.8. Retinoblastoma. Section of an eye excised for advanced retinoblastoma; this is seen to be half-filling the vitreous cavity, and extending up the optic nerve which is strikingly swollen; the lens has become cataractous and dislocated, while neoplastic cells largely fill the anterior chamber. (From the museum at the Institute of Ophthalmology.)

* An eye may need to be removed in order to save life, sight or pain; in other words—(1) for malignant tumours; (2) if sympathetic ophthalmitis threatens; (3) if it is blind and painful; in the last group an attempt is usually made simply to relieve the pain by a retrobulbar injection of alcohol, unless the globe is purulent, ruptured or disfiguring.

CHAPTER 6

THE INJURED EYE

Although the overhanging orbital ridges afford great protection against direct injury from any large object, small particles notoriously find their way into the eye, with effects which are disproportionately irritating in the case of corneal foreign bodies, or damaging in the case of perforating wounds.

CONTUSION OF THE EYE

The following lesions may be caused:

Haematoma of eyelids

The classical 'black eye': blood oozes freely into the loose subcutaneous tissues, and then lingers there for about two weeks. Apart from an inspection of the eyeball to exclude further damage, no treatment is necessary.

Subconjunctival haemorrhage (Plate 12, following p. 60).

This usually involves only one sector and does not appear to extend backwards into the orbital tissues (if there is no such limitation posteriorly, it may be a forward extension from an intra-orbital haemorrhage, and so may signify a fracture of the skull that involves the orbital walls). The large majority of these haemorrhages are spontaneous, especially in arteriosclerotics, or less commonly are due to a sudden venous congestion as in whooping cough. They are symptomless, and, again, take about two weeks to disperse.

Corneal abrasion

The epithelium is readily stripped off the corneal surface, often over a large area, leaving a very painful, irritable eye. The abrasion may be difficult to see, unless an irregularity is noticed of the corneal light-reflections (as from the window), but it can easily be demonstrated by inserting a vital stain such as fluorescein which renders the denuded area bright green. The epithelium quickly regenerates, provided the eyelids are kept closed by a pad and bandage (to splint the cornea, and at the same time relieve pain and photophobia), and the abrasion remains uninfected (antibiotic ointment should be inserted to prevent the abrasion turning into a corneal ulcer). Such healed abrasions occasionally re-open spontaneously many months later ('recurrent abrasions').

The iris

Contusions frequently cause a little *bleeding* into the anterior chamber—a 'hyphaema', blood gravitating to the lower segment, and dispersing a few days later; only if the whole anterior chamber is filled with blood is there a danger that the aqueous drainage may be obstructed, and the resultant secondary glaucoma will then require surgical relief (incision at the corneal margin so that the blood can be evacuated). However, even small traumatic hyphaemas should be treated by bed-rest, as a major secondary haemorrhage may follow some days later. Major *tears* may occur at the iris root (an 'iridodialysis', the pupil then becoming D-shaped) or at the sphincter; and even without a visible tear, the sphincter may be paralysed for some weeks, or even permanently, as a 'traumatic mydriasis'. These tears show little attempt at healing, but rarely interfere with sight. Atropine drops are sometimes prescribed until the eye is quiet.

The lens

A *concussion cataract* may form, similar to that induced by heat or radiation, and merit removal. *Dislocations* are usually partial, so that the lens is drawn to one side with consequent visual distortion; occasionally the suspensory ligament is completely broken, and the lens falls backwards into the vitreous (leaving a tremulous, unsupported iris—an 'iridodonesis'), or slips through the pupil into the anterior chamber (inducing a painful spasm of the pupil behind it, and a secondary glaucoma by obstructing the aqueous drainage). Partial dislocations of the lens are sometimes found as a bilateral congenital mishap, often in association with arachnodactyly and other systemic defects, and again betrayed by a tremulous pupil margin.

The retina

Contusions of the eyeball may cause a transient retinal *anaesthesia* (a 'black-out'), without objective changes. More severe blows may cause retinal oedema which is ophthalmoscopically visible as a whitish cloud obscuring the red fundus pattern; this normally clears in a few days, but may leave a little residue of pigment proliferation with an equivalent scotoma of depressed vision. A localised oedema is typically found at the macula, similar to that caused by infra-red rays, in 'eclipse-blindness'.

Retinal *haemorrhages* generally remain small, and cause visual embarrassment only if overlying the macula; occasionally they irrupt into the vitreous where the loss of vision may be almost complete, and with the ophthalmoscope the red fundus reflex is correspondingly almost or completely obscured. The latter take many months to clear, and if extensive or repeated, the clot may organize and permanently impair the sight. *Tears* usually occur at the anterior limit of the retina, and may lead to a retinal detachment, which spreads across the macular area some weeks later. Sometimes only the choroid is ruptured, causing a white streak (of exposed sclera) in the fundus, usually near the disc or macula.

Optic nerve

The optic nerve may be torn or compressed in fractures involving the orbital walls, and blindness is usually immediate, complete and permanent, the dense pallor of a primary optic atrophy becoming ophthalmoscopically visible several weeks later.

PERFORATING INJURIES

Wounds of the eyelids require prompt suturing, with exact restoration of the torn lid margin; the blood supply of the lids is so profuse that such lacerations heal well and hardly ever become infected. If the lower lacrimal canaliculus is torn, it must be re-united over a splint to prevent a permanent barrier to the drainage of tears. Conjunctival lacerations require suturing only if they are very extensive, as they heal rapidly.

Burns of the eyelids are more serious because of the risk of subsequent distortion of the lids with cicatrization (entropion or ectropion), and hence of corneal ulceration through exposure. The treatment entails inspection of the eyeball, which must be carefully examined to exclude further damage and to remove any foreign bodies, followed by instillation of atropine and antibiotic ointment, before the reactionary oedema renders the lids difficult to separate. The skin should be dusted with sulphona-mide-penicillin powder, and further routine measures may be needed if the burns are extensive. In the case of chemical burns, the eye should be copiously irrigated, as by immersing the head promptly in a basin of water; while with alkali burns the risk of a subsequent symblepharon will command further attention.

Perforating wounds of **cornea** or **sclera** are often small and barely visible, but they should be suspected if the history is suggestive and any intra-ocular lesion is apparent. Perforating wounds require surgical closure if they are gaping, and since the iris will generally have fallen forwards to plug any corneal wound through which the aqueous has escaped (Plate 13, following p. 60), this 'prolapsed' iris must first be excised, before the wound is closed. As immediate treatment, atropine and antibiotic drops should be instilled.

The presence of a retained foreign body must first be excluded—a special liability after the use of a hammer and chisel. Sometimes such foreign bodies are visible; and they can usually be demonstrated radiographically, or signalled by a sharp pain when they are shifted in the field of a giant magnet. Small particles that have sufficient force to penetrate the tough wall of the eyeball are generally metallic and then usually magnetic, so that they can be extracted with the giant magnet, otherwise their evacuation may be difficult and hazardous.

Retained iron particles will gradually dissolve, but the brown pigment is then dispersed through the intra-ocular tissues ('siderosis bulbi'), and the sight is gradually destroyed. Other metals tend to provoke suppuration; while some foreign bodies, like glass, may remain inert for years.

Perforating injuries to the **lens** will disrupt the lens capsule and cause a cataract.

Pyogenic infection of the eyeball often follows such injuries, and pus can be seen to accumulate in the anterior chamber as a hypopyon. The inflammation generally recedes, leaving a shrunken, blind eye—'phthisis bulbi'; but the pus may spread into the scleral lamellae, and the globe finally rupture. These cases need antibiotic therapy, systemically and by subconjunctival injection; but when a panophthalmitis is established, little hope remains of saving the eye, and the pain and toxaemia lend an urgency to its removal. This is normally performed by an 'evisceration' in which the disorganized contents are scooped away from the scleral envelope (the latter being left behind to prevent the risk of disseminating infection into the orbital contents, and up through the sheath of the optic nerve). In other circumstances the eye is removed by an 'enucleation' (Fig. 6.1) in which the conjunctiva is divided by a circular sweep over the rectus insertions, which are then themselves cut, allowing the eyeball to be prolapsed, and the optic nerve to be reached and divided. Sympathetic ophthalmitis has been noted as an occasional devastating sequel to perforating wounds, especially when they involve the ciliary region and are not purulent; and the injured eye may need to be removed if the inflammation

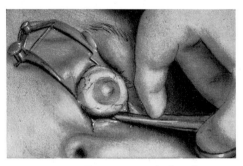

Fig. 6.1. Enucleation of the eye. The rectus muscles have been severed, and the optic nerve is being divided with scissors, after dislocating the eyeball forwards between the blades of the speculum. (May and Worth's *Diseases of the Eye*.)

shows little improvement after three weeks, as a prophylactic against involvement of its fellow eye. Otherwise the eye is excised only if grossly disorganized, or blind and persistently painful.

Non-perforating foreign bodies generally become impacted on the cornea where they provoke a characteristic irritation, augmented by every movement of the eyelid. They should be removed (after anaesthetizing the cornea with a drop of amethocaine); a piece of cotton-wool will occasionally suffice for this if they are very superficial, but usually they need to be excavated with a flattened needle (a blunt 'Spud', that simply hammers the projecting end of the embedded particle, is still frequently preferred from timidity, ignorance or habit). Thereafter antibiotic ointment should be inserted, with atropine (1 per cent) if the crater is deep and the eye very irritable; and the lid should be kept closed with an eye-pad until the epithelium has healed. If no foreign body can be seen on the cornea, the upper lid should be everted (Fig. 1.3) as such particles are frequently caught in a horizontal groove beneath the tarsus, where they abrade the cornea with each blink, and whence they can easily be whisked away with the ball of the finger.

BLOW-OUT FRACTURES

Fractures of the orbit are fairly common sequels to facial injury, they are associated almost inevitably with marked ecchymosis and subconjunctival haemorrhage (which has no evident posterior limitation), and occasionally with crepitus if a sinus has been opened, as well as other localizing signs; these fractures are readily recognized on routine X-ray, and heal without active intervention.

A blow on the eyeball may, however, cause such a rise in intra-orbital pressure that the orbital contents are forced through the thin orbital floor, and so herniate into the antrum (exceptionally into the ethmoidal air-cells). Such 'Blow-out fractures' are easily overlooked, since the initial bruising may at first neutralize the tell-tale enophthalmos; but this develops later, along with an evident tethering of the eyeball, when the muscles (usually inferior rectus and oblique) become trapped in the hernia, limiting elevation of the eye and causing diplopia.

A straight X-ray may fail to show up the fracture, but there may be a unilateral opacity of the antrum from haemorrhage, or it may contain a hammock-like shadow, suspended from the orbital floor. A loss of sensation over the intra-orbital nerve distribution may be diagnostic.

Minor derangements—without diplopia—are rare and need no correction, but if diplopia is still present after two weeks, the herniated orbital contents should be gently elevated, and the gap closed by a bone graft or a sheet of silicone rubber.

CHAPTER 7
REFRACTIVE ERRORS

The normal eye is so shaped that rays of light from a distant object are made to converge on traversing the convex corneal and lens surfaces, and are brought to an exact focus on the retina. Nearer objects can then be brought into focus by a contraction of the ciliary muscle allowing the lens to become more spherical.

There are four types of 'refractive error' in which the images are not focused correctly on the retina: the inadequacy of accommodation that comes in middle-age (Presbyopia), variations in the length of the eyeball (Hypermetropia and Myopia), and variations in the corneal curvatures between different meridians (Astigmatism). These may all be remedied by appropriately-curved spectacle lenses. A pinhole aperture will also neutralise the blurring caused by a refractive error; and this provides a useful test to indicate whether a poor visual acuity is simply due to such an optical distortion rather than an organic impediment to sight.

Presbyopia

The range of focusing (or 'accommodation') decreases throughout life as the lens becomes stiffer with age, so that the nearest point that can be brought into focus on the retina recedes beyond the normal reading-range at about the age of 45, and presbyopia is then said to have set in. This can be compensated by weak convex reading spectacles, which will require strengthening every few years.

Hypermetropia

For the *Short* eyeball, distant objects can be brought to a focus on the retina, which here lies in front of the normal focal point, by using a convex spectacle lens (Fig. 7.1). In the youthful hypermetrope such a focusing is normally done spontaneously by accommodating the lens of the eye, but this leaves less reserve of focusing for near-vision, so that fatigue-symptoms on near-work may develop (usually in adolescence), or a decreasing

DISTANCE   NEAR

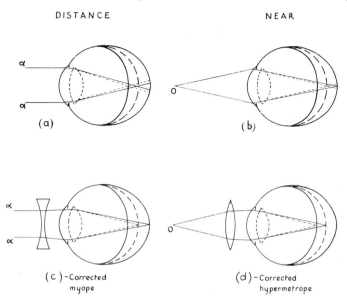

(a)   (b)

(C) -Corrected   (d) -Corrected
   myope   hypermetrope

Fig. 7.1. Refraction in the hypermetropic and myopic eye. The continuous lines represent the short (hypermetropic) and the long (myopic) eyeballs, and the intermediate (interrupted) line represents the normal-lengthed, normal-sighted eye. The effect of accommodation in bringing forward the point of focus is shown by the dotted line.

The posterior principal focus, which falls onto the retina in the normal-lengthed eyeball both in distance-vision (*a*) and near-vision + accommodation (*b*), only falls onto the hypermetropic retina when the eye is accommodated alone (*a*), and onto the myopic retina only during near-vision in the absence of accommodation (*b*).

(*c*) shows the myope, with his concave spectacle lens pushing his focal point backwards towards his backward-placed retina, so as to allow clear distance-vision.

(*d*) shows the hypermetrope, with his convex spectacle lens bringing his focal point forwards towards his forward-placed retina so as to allow clear near-vision.

near-range of vision may be encountered before the usual age of 45. These merit the assistance of convex spectacle lenses for close work (Fig. 7.1*d*).

Myopia

For the *Long* eyeball, distant objects can only be brought to a focus on a retina, which here lies behind the normal focal point, by a concave spectacle lens (Fig. 7.1*c*). However, near objects can still be focused on the retinal by inhibiting the normal reflex of accommodation (Fig. 7.1*b*), myopes are thus 'short-sighted'. In the large majority of cases the myopia is simply a physiological variant of length, as is hypermetropia; it ceases to progress after adolescence, and a little reduction of the myopia may even follow in late middle-age. In a minority of cases the eyeball may continue to elongate throughout life ('progressive myopia') leading to a retinal degeneration (Plate 14, following p. 60), or even detachment.

It may here be noted that myopic eyeballs often do, in fact, look large, even exophthalmic; and through the ophthalmoscope the optic disc in myopia seems proportionately large and pale—simulating an optic atrophy (Plate 7(*d*), following p. 60), whereas the optic disc in hypermetropia looks small and pink—often simulating a papilloedema ('pseudo-papilloedema'), (Plate 7(*f*), following p. 60).

Astigmatism

Here the eyeball is flattened, generally from above downwards, but sometimes sideways, or along an oblique axis. Vision is then proportionately blurred both for near and distance, irrespective of accommodation, and visual fatigue (ocular headaches) may occasionally accrue. In the rare cases where the astigmatism is sufficient to cause symptoms, these can be compensated by spectacle lenses with an appropriately different curvature in the two meridians.

TESTING OF REFRACTION

Performed either subjectively (finding by trial-and-error which lens gives best visual acuity, and ordering the strongest convex lens or weakest concave lens that permits full vision) or objectively (determining by 'retinoscopy' what strength of lens is required to neutralize the movement of a beam of light reflected from the fundus); this latter technique requires considerable practice, but is more secure than the subjective method, and is the only way of refracting the woolly-minded adult or inarticulate child. Such a retinoscopy can only be accurate if the ciliary muscle is at rest; so a mydriatic should first be instilled, and for the powerful ciliary muscles of children repeated applications of atropine are usually needed.

SPECTACLES

Spectacles are thus required either to improve visual acuity, or else to relieve an 'eye-strain' or headaches (but only when such symptoms may be legitimately attributed to the particular refractive error that is present), and such spectacles should be used therafter only if they materially improve the vision or specifically relieve these fatigue-symptoms. It must be emphasized that the vast majority of headaches bear no relationship to refractive errors, and also that the eyes themselves can never be damaged by uncorrected or wrongly-corrected refractive errors.* Refractive errors are due to anatomical variations, and the progress of myopia is likewise genetically determined, so that refractive errors cannot be remedied or their progress curbed by medicaments, diet, exercise, or any other fanciful nostra.

Spectacle lenses are thus convex (for presbyopia or hypermetropia) or concave (for myopia); and since the curve of the cornea is rarely exactly the same in all meridians, this associated astigmatism (generally too slight to demand treatment of itself) is then also corrected by giving the spectacle lens an added convexity or concavity in the appropriate meridian. The strength or 'power' of such lenses is measured in terms of dioptres (1 'D' = 1/focal length of the lens in metres). Finally, a prism can be incorporated into such lenses to compensate a slight malalignment of the eyes ('latent squint'), but this is, in fact, hardly ever indicated. Spectacle lenses can be darkened, like sun-glasses, and very occasionally a genuine photophobia justifies this, but the vast majority of dark glasses are sought in the hope of protecting a frail psyche or concealing a guiltful one from the harsh or revealing light of day.

Contact lenses are spectacle lenses that slip beneath the eye-lids and thus are barely visible externally. These are optically necessary for the very rare cases of corneal irregularity, optically useful for high myopia, and uniocular aphakia, and cosmetically convenient for the low myopes who count their glasses a social blemish. Nowadays the majority of lenses provided are the small 'corneals', fitted readily (albeit often expensively) *hard* from stock, and well tolerated for most of the day. The larger soft *soft (porous)* ('hydrophilic') lenses cause even less discomfort, but are more clumsy, fragile, less readily sterilized and more expensive. The still larger 'haptic' *haptic* lenses, the earliest form, which were moulded to fit over the anterior scleral curvature, are now restricted to therapeutic or protective uses.

---

* The only occasion where glasses may help to prevent impairment of sight is in some rare cases of amblyopia in small children, where the suppression of function is central rather than ocular (in small squinting children they may also help the development of binocularity). In all other cases spectacles are justified only when they sufficiently improve the vision or comfort to outweigh their nuisance-value.

CHAPTER 8
SQUINT AND NYSTAGMUS

[handwritten: paralytic   concomitant]

Squint (or 'Strabismus') means a deviation of the eyes* so that their axes are no longer parallel, but excluding the normal convergence that accompanies near-vision. Deviations may be in any direction, but are most commonly horizontal (convergent or divergent). Such a deviation of the visual axes is obvious if the squint is gross; but small degrees of squint can be recognised from the asymmetrical positions of the bright corneal light-reflections relative to their respective pupil margins, and confirmed by covering each eye in turn, and noting whether a perceptible movement is made by either eye to assume fixation, when its fellow-eye is occluded.

The eyes are kept parallel by a complicated conditioned reflex, acquired during the first few years of life in the interests of single vision; this reflex is consolidated when the child learns to fuse the two superimposed images (from either eye) and finally to appreciate stereoscopic vision.

The squint is labelled *paralytic* if the motor-apparatus that rotates the eye is damaged. It is labelled *concomitant* if there is an impediment to the sensory component of the reflex arc (e.g. a poor-sighted eye from any cause) or to the central component of the reflex arc (e.g. mental deficiency, psychic disturbance). Such a concomitant squint, in which the visual axes deviate at a constant angle irrespective of the direction of gaze, is the commonest squint of childhood. As these children are usually hypermetropic, and the squint is often hereditary, the underlying cause in most cases would appear to be some genetic impediment to binocularity, aggravated by the extra accommodation (with its associated convergence) that is required in such a hypermetropic eye (p. 76).

[handwritten marginalia: anatomical poor vision / barinmatic / hypermetropia]

[handwritten: short-eye ball : blurred short vision ie long-sighted]

PARALYTIC SQUINT

SIGNS AND SYMPTOMS

The affected eye will have *limited movement* in the direction of the action of the paralysed muscle; the *angle of deviation* will thus be greatest in that

---

* The word 'squint' is sometimes carelessly and erroneously used to signify a half-closure of the eyes, or the inspection of objects at a very close range.

direction, and the *double-vision* that results will similarly be greatest in that same direction.

The secondary signs include an *alteration of posture*: thus a paralysed left lateral rectus will cause an increasing squint and increasing double-vision ('diplopia') on looking to the left, but on looking to the right the left lateral rectus will not be needed, and the visual axes will become parallel; the patient thus learns to avoid diplopia by turning his head to the left and looking out of the right-hand corner of his eyes. Similarly a tilt of the head laterally or forwards (Fig. 8.1) may compensate for weakness of one of the vertically-acting muscles (requiring differentiation from the other forms of torticollis).

Paralysis of the lateral and medial recti produces a simple horizontal deviation of the eyes and horizontal diplopia. The line of action of the other extra-ocular muscles is more complex (Fig. 8.2). Since the superior and inferior recti take origin at the orbital apex, which is well medial to the eyeball's centre of rotation, both will tend to adduct the eye, as well as elevating and depressing it (respectively); only when the eye is directed laterally (*abducted*) so that it lies along the axis of these rectus muscles do the latter act as pure elevators or depressors; and when the eye is already *adducted*, so that it is directed almost perpendicular to their axis, these rectus muscles act almost entirely as adductors (Fig. 8.3). Similarly the two oblique muscles have a secondary effect of abducting, which is most

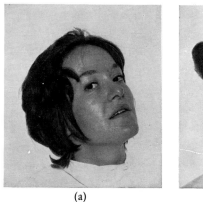 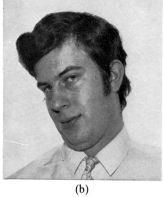

(a)   (b)

Fig. 8.1. Ocular torticollis. Examples of compensating postures: (*a*) Face turned to L., head tilted to R., chin elevated—to compensate for Left Supr. Rectus palsy. (*b*) Face turned to R., head tilted to R., chin depressed—to compensate for Left Supr. Oblique palsy.

Recti — elev supp } when abd. Add when add.

Obliques — elev supp } when add. Abd when abd.

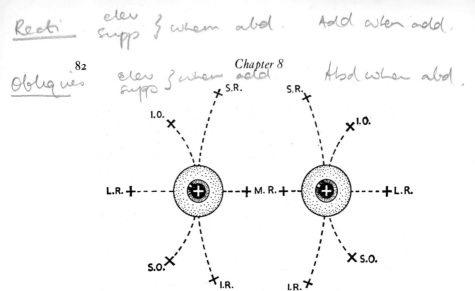

Fig. 8.2. The line of action of the individual extra-ocular muscles, showing also their torsional effects, and indicating the various contralateral synergists (S.R.+I.O., I.R.+S.O., M.R.+L.R.).

marked when the eyes are already abducted; while they act almost entirely as elevators (the inferior obliques) and depressors (the superior obliques) when the eye is adducted and lies nearly along their line of action—running from the anteromedial corners of the orbit to insert at the back of the eye on its outer aspect (Fig. 8.3). These vertical muscles thus act in concert, the superior rectus and inferior oblique collaborating to elevate the eye (neutralizing each other's secondary effects of abduction and adduction), while the superior and inferior recti will both assist the medial rectus in adducting the eye, and neutralizing each other's vertical pull. A further complication of these four vertically-acting muscles is their tertiary effect in 'torsion'—rolling the eye about an antero-posterior axis (thus the superior rectus rolls the top of the eye over towards the nose, causing an 'intorsion'); these effects are similarly neutralized by the collaboration of different muscles in each ocular movement, aided by the synergistic muscles of the fellow eye.

ASSESSMENT

The limitation of movement may be obvious and promptly indicate the affected muscle (Fig. 8.4). The diplopia, which is usually of sudden onset, disappears on covering either eye; and the more blurred and more displaced image will belong to the affected eye. The palsied muscles can be

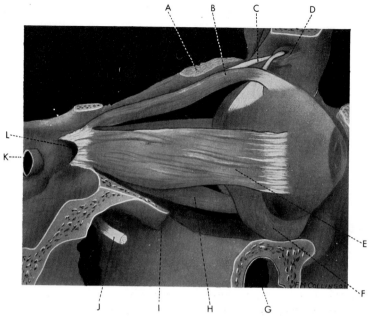

Fig. 8.3. Anatomy of the extra-ocular muscles from the lateral aspect. (A) Levator Palpebrae Superioris Muscle; (B) Superior Rectus Muscle; (C) Superior Oblique Muscle; (D) Pulley; (E) Lateral Rectus Muscle; (F) Inferior Oblique Muscle; (G) Maxillary Antrum; (H) Inferior Rectus Muscle; (I) Inferior Orbital Fissure; (J) Maxillary Nerve (Vb); (K) Internal Carotid Artery; (L) Optic Foramen. (Wolff, *Anatomy of the Eye and Orbit*.)

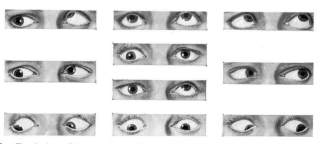

Fig. 8.4. Deviation of the eyes in paralysis of the R. superior rectus, in each of the nine cardinal directions of gaze. The two central pictures show the deviation on looking straight ahead, the upper one when the left eye is fixing, and the lower one when the right eye is fixing. (Duke-Elder, *Textbook of Ophthalmology*.)

identified by noting in which of the nine positions of gaze the diplopia is worst, and the eye from which the respective images are derived can be distinguished by the wearing of different coloured goggles (Fig. 8.5).

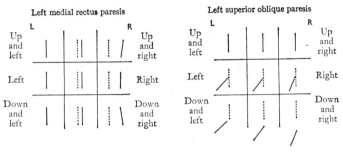

Fig. 8.5. The assessment of Diplopia by charting the doubled images, in the case of paresis of (*a*) left medial rectus, and (*b*) left superior oblique. The patient wears a red glass in front of the right eye, and the dotted line shows the position of this right-eye's image.

AETIOLOGY

Any cause of nerve or muscle damage may be responsible. The common causes include: trauma (to brain or orbit), vascular disease (e.g. aneurysm of circle of Willis, intra-orbital or intra-cranial haemorrhage, or thrombosis of the nutrient vessels to the individual nerves), neuritis (e.g. disseminated sclerosis or syphilis), metabolic (e.g. dysthyroid exophthalmos), cerebral tumour, etc.

TREATMENT

Any evident underlying disease must first have attention. The diplopia may then be relieved—most simply by occluding the deviating eye (e.g. by tissue-paper gummed on its spectacle lens); while in an established paralysis surgery to the extra-ocular muscles can at least render the eyes straight when looking directly forwards, and discordant eye movements can then be largely avoided by movement of the head rather than the eyes.

CONCOMITANT SQUINT

Here the eyes adopt an abnormal position in relation to one another—usually of convergence, but the complicated yoking of the eye movements (through reciprocal innervations) serves to keep this angle of deviation constant in all directions of gaze. Such a concomitant squint normally develops during the first few years of life, before the reflex of binocular vision has had time to become established; and, when it has not been induced at an earlier age from some organic impediment to vision (e.g. a congenital cataract), it is often precipitated when illness or emotional travail so depletes the child's energies that he can no longer make the subconscious effort to keep the eyes straight. In such cases the infant's eyes generally exhibit their natural tendency to converge; (infants are long-sighted, and this entails an excess of accommodation; but, as the 'near-reflex' is a synkinesis involving accommodation, convergence and pupillary constriction, each one of these movements tends automatically to induce the other two).

Infants can quickly learn to suppress the vision of a squinting eye, to avoid the diplopia that such a deviation must first induce; and if this suppression is maintained for several years, it may become impossible to counteract, so that the eye remains permanently poor-sighted—an '*amblyopia*', or, more familiarly, a 'lazy eye'. Sometimes the child learns to suppress the vision of either eye at will, so that both eyes retain good vision but cannot be used in unison—an 'alternating concomitant convergent squint'. As age advances there is an increasing tendency for eyes to diverge, thus convergent concomitant squints do tend to straighten later (a 'natural cure'), although usually at the expense of an amblyopic eye; while eyes which become blinded in adult life similarly tend to swing outwards sooner or later.

TREATMENT

The first essential is that all cases of suspected squint should be referred promptly for examination by an eye-surgeon. The squint may be the first evidence of other disorders (such as a retinoblastoma), it may be only a 'pseudosquint' due to wide epicanthic folds (and the parents can then be reassured), and if it is a true squint it is necessary to prevent the development of amblyopia before it is too late. When the child is too young to test, ambylopia can usually be assumed, in an eye which constantly squints and maintains fixation poorly, and rectified by *occluding* the better-seeing eye (Fig. 8.6), thus forcing the child to use the squinting eye; this is usually successful before the age of 7 but rarely after the age of 10. The underlying tendency to converge should then be neutralized by correcting any hypermetropia with appropriate convex *spectacles* (infants are very rarely myopic,

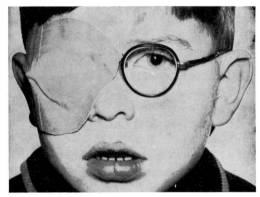

Fig. 8.6. Occlusion of the better-seeing eye in squint. The simplest method is by fixing two layers of Elastoplast over the spectacle lens, and trimming this to fit the patient's face.

but in such cases there will be a corresponding tendency to develop a divergent squint). If a marked squint persists in spite of correct glasses and the prevention of amblyopia, an *operation* is usually indicated to re-align the squinting eye (Fig. 8.7); this normally entails the reinsertion of the medial rectus tendon farther back on the globe (a 'recession') and an equivalent shortening of the lateral rectus tendon (a 'resection'), for the common convergent squint. By about the age of 5 the child can also collaborate in *orthoptic exercises*. These are sensory exercises that help the eyes to build up their fusion and ultimately their stereoscopic vision (and not exercises for the eye-muscles, as the patient usually imagines); such exercises will rarely cure a squint, but the presence of full binocular vision

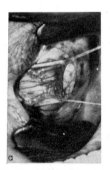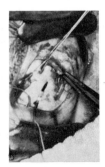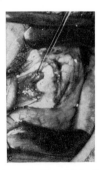

Fig. 8.7. Recession of lateral rectus. (*a*) Sutures placed through either edge of exposed muscle. (*b*) Muscle divided at insertion, and sutures being inserted through sclera, 5 mm behind this. (*c*) Suturing completed.

will always help to keep straight those eyes which spectacles or operation have brought into rough alignment. Squinting eyes can always be brought straight by an operation at any age for cosmetic effect, but they may well drift out of alignment later, as there will be no further development of binocular vision, and no significant return of vision in an amblyopic eye over the age of 10. Because of the rapid decline of the child's capacity to recover suppressed vision and to achieve full binocularity, it is particularly important that all squinting children should have specialist advice as soon as the squint is noted.

Latent squint

This signifies a tendency to squint which has usually developed after the child has acquired enough binocular vision to hold the eyes in alignment for most of the time, and only when the objects presented to the two eyes are different, or fatigue prevails, does a concomitant squint become manifest. Such latent squints can very occasionally be relieved by prismatic glasses, sometimes they even need an operative correction, but generally they cause no symptoms and require no active treatment. A small degree of horizontal latent squint is indeed present in most healthy eyes.

NYSTAGMUS

These oscillations of the eyes may be ocular or labyrinthine-cerebellar in origin.

The *ocular nystagmus* has regular pendulum-like movements, which are exaggerated on looking to either side; the movements are generally horizontal, but may have a vertical or rotatory component. Such a pendular nystagmus develops in infants who cannot obtain a clear image on their maculas, either because of some bilateral physical impediment (such as a congenital cataract or corneal opacity, or a less obvious defect such as retinal damage or optic atrophy), or the dazzle from extraneous light (as in albinos), or an idiopathic 'congenital nystagmus' without any evident cause, but with poor central vision in consequence.

The *labyrinthine-cerebellar* nystagmus has movements that show a slow drift in one direction and a fast correcting jerk back again; the direction of the nystagmus is conventionally labelled according to the direction of the fast (correcting) phase. The slower drift is generally towards the side of the lesion (e.g. middle-ear damage, acoustic neuroma), and the movements are usually exaggerated on looking in the opposite direction.

A rather indefinite, 'wobbling', nystagmus is particularly common in multiple sclerosis.

Internal ophthalmoplegia

A palsy of the iris and ciliary muscles usually reflects damage to their sympathetic or parasympathetic nerve supply; but an intracranial haemorrhage may be disclosed by pupil contraction from irritation (first, on the affected site only), followed by dilatation from the paralysis of the sphincter.

The *Argyll Robertson* pupil, with a loss of direct and indirect light reflexes but retention of the near reflex, probably results from a lesion in the mid-brain. Such pupils are small, irregular and usually unequal; they dilate poorly with atropine and constrict promptly on accommodation; although a characteristic feature of tabes (about 70 per cent), they are also found in about half the cases of general paralysis of the insane, and in a variety of other toxic and inflammatory lesions of the brain stem.

The *myoyonic pupil* (*Adie's pupil*) superficially resembles the Argyll Robertson pupil, but is most frequently found in young women. The myotonic pupil is larger then normal, and therefore larger than its fellow since it is usually uniocular; there is a very slow and protracted constriction on near vision, and an even more sluggish constriction with light; it dilates fully with atropine, and there may be other signs of associated nervous damage, such as absent knee and ankle jerks. The cause is unknown and there is no effective treatment.

Horner's syndrome. Damage to the cervical sympathetic will cause the triad of miosis, partial ptosis and enophthalmos, from weakening of the various sympathetic-innervated muscles of the orbit. This syndrome may result from a host of lesions, such as cervical adenitis, operations on the thyroid, and aortic aneurysms. It is also found in *syringomyelia*, due to a distension of the central canal of the spinal cord in the lower cervical and thoracic region.

CHAPTER 9
THE CENTRAL MECHANISM OF VISION

The **optic nerve** is essentially an isthmus of central nervous tissue, consisting almost exclusively of the fibres from the ganglion cells of the retina, conveying information from the rods and cones to the lateral geniculate bodies. At the optic chiasma the fibres which lie in the medial half of the nerve cross over and continue backwards in the optic tract of the opposite side, which winds around the cerebral peduncles, accompanied by the posterior cerebral vessels. From the lateral geniculate body the second nerve-fibre relay sweeps back as the optic radiations to reach an area of the occipital cortex, which includes its tip and the adjacent medial surface. Here the visual image is crystallized, with each point geographically corresponding to a point on each retina; and from this image the conscious 'percept' is derived.

In their long journey backwards these fibre-relays may be damaged by a wide miscellany of lesions—traumatic, vascular, inflammatory and neoplastic, all of which may be disclosed by specific encroachments of the visual fields. So it is of especial importance to know the relative positions of the various fibre-bundles at each level (Fig. 9.1); and if the lesion lies anterior to the geniculate bodies there will also be immediately recognizable changes in the optic nerve head—oedema or atrophy.

Papilloedema (Plate 7e, following p. 60)

An oedema of the nerve head ('papilla') elevates the disc forward from the retina, tends to fill in the central (physiological) optic pit, and blurs the disc margins. Along with this comes a venous engorgement that makes the disc redder than normal and often spattered with small haemorrhages.

It is generally due to pressure on the central retinal vein, as this crosses the sleeve of arachnoid and cerebro-spinal fluid which extends forwards around the optic nerve as far as the eyeball, and so transmits any rise of intracranial pressure; hence it is usually the first diagnostic sign of a cerebral tumour. In such cases, the visual acuity is unaffected, but a check of the central field will show an enlargement of the blind-spot correspond-

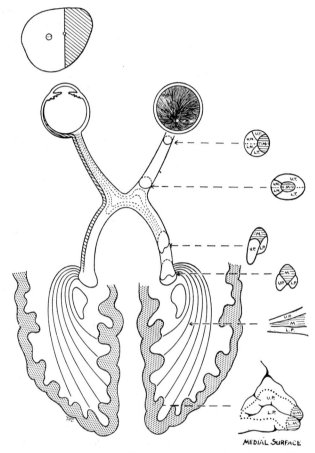

Fig. 9.1. Localization in the Visual Pathways. Showing distribution of fibres-prechiasmal (macular, upper and lower nasal and temporal) and retro-chiasmal (macular, upper and lower peripheral).

ing to the distribution of the disc oedema. Occasionally, the disc oedema is simply part of a generalized retinal oedema (as in the case of malignant hypertension—Plate 9, following p. 60) or of a focal inflammation (a 'papillitis'), in which case there is always a gross visual loss.

Optic atrophy

An atrophy of the optic nerve fibres is revealed by a pallor of the disc, due to an atrophy of their supporting capillaries. This may be due to a primary damage to the nerve fibres—a *simple optic atrophy* (Plate 7*h*, following p. 60), or else it may follow a papilloedema, when it is styled a *post-neuritic optic atrophy* (Plate 7*g*, following p.60), and the disc margins and central pit then seem less well-defined, with glial tissue also sheathing the emergent vessels. A third group is the *consecutive optic atrophy*, following damage to the parent ganglion cells of the retina (as in choroido-retinitis, dystrophies or central artery occlusion).

The differential diagnosis of a pale disc may be difficult, since physiological variations in colour are great, and the disc is naturally pale in both infancy and old age, as is also the enlarged disc of a myopic eye; and where only a few fibre bundles are damaged (as in multiple sclerosis) the change of colour may be slight.

The *aetiology* of simple optic atrophy covers many local and systemic disorders among which the most common may be listed as follows:

(*a*) Trauma—severance or avulsion of the optic nerve, in which the blindness is immediate and the atrophy complete, or compression by fractures around the orbital apex. Even mild injuries occasionally cause an optic atrophy, presumably from intraneural haemorrhage.

Where the loss of sight is incomplete, the site of the damage can usually be pin-pointed by relating the area of visual field destroyed to the position of these fibres in the optic pathways (Fig. 9.2).

(*b*) Compression—this may be due to aneurysms, bony over-growth (as oxycephaly and Paget's disease), or, less certainly, adhesions (as in basal arachnoiditis); but a partial optic atrophy due to compression most commonly derives from a pituitary tumour, provoking a bitemporal hemianopia, which usually starts as an erosion of the upper temporal fields (since the tumour arises from below—Fig. 9.3), and often mainly on one side (since the tumour is usually asymmetrical).

(*c*) Ischaemic atrophy—arterial occlusion, anaemia, glaucoma.

(*d*) Post-inflammatory atrophy—the spread of an adjacent inflammation (such as meningitis), or part of a generalized central nervous infection, as disseminated sclerosis, in which the central fibres of the optic nerve are damaged, leaving a paracentral scotoma (Fig. 9.4), and tabes, in which the loss is mainly peripheral (Fig. 9.5).

(*e*) Toxic atrophy ('toxic amblyopia'). In the majority of forms the optic nerve-fibres from the central area are affected, producing a central or paracentral scotoma, and they are often accompanied by signs of a peripheral neuritis elsewhere; the minority (including those caused by organic arsenic and tabes) depress vision generally, so that the impulses from the

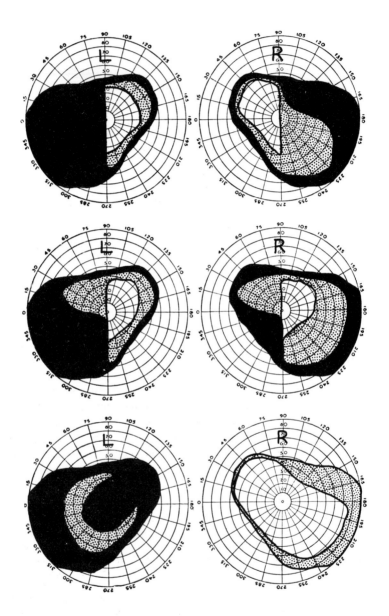

Optic Nerves

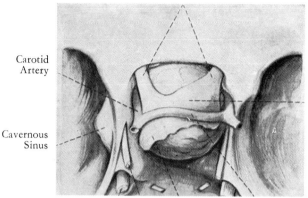

Carotid
Artery

Chiasma

Cavernous
Sinus

V   III   Optic Tract   Antr. Comm. Art.

Fig. 9.3. Pituitary Tumour, compressing the lower fibres of the chiasma. The chiasma is seen to be compressed by the underlying tumour (which is extending into the left middle fossa) with the anterior communicating artery stretched over it. (Duke-Elder.)

less sensitive retinal periphery become submerged, and the visual fields show a peripheral constriction (Fig. 9.5). These poisons include cyanide from tobacco, methyl and ethyl alcohol, quinine, lead and arsenic; although presenting as an optic atrophy from axon degeneration, the damage is probably inflicted on the parent cells of these axons—the ganglion cells of the retina. The visual loss may be acute if large amounts of the poison are ingested, as with methyl alcohol and quinine, but it is usually insidious, as in the commonest form—the tobacco amblyopia which follows prolonged and heavy use of cheap pipe tobacco. The latter is a composite disorder, partly due to dietary deficiency (especially of vitamin B); this is aggravated by alcohol and an associated megaloblastic anaemia, and particularly by the presence of cyanide from tobacco smoke, which a deficiency of B_{12} renders less readily detoxified. Abstinence is the essential treatment, combined with adequate doses of vitamine B_{12}.

Fig. 9.2. Field defects from lesions of the optic pathways. (*a*) Bitemporal hemianopia, resulting from a pituitary tumour. The loss initially affects only the upper quadrants; in this case vision in the right lower quadrant has yet to be destroyed. (*b*) Homonymous hemianopia. Lower left quadrantic hemianopia from a right upper tract lesion. (*c*) Field loss due to a prechiasmal aneurysm, pressing on the left optic nerve (with early loss of the macular fibres), but extending far enough back towards the chiasma to involve the lower crossed nasal fibres from the other eye.

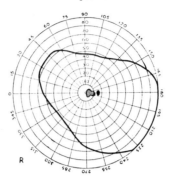

Fig. 9.4. Paracentral scotoma, as in tobacco amblyopia.

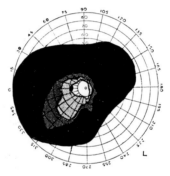

Fig. 9.5. Peripheral field loss as in tabes.

(*f*) Malnutrition, especially the lack of vitamin B, may damage the ganglion cells directly, or indirectly through retinal ischaemia.

(*g*) Degenerative diseases—atrophy may accompany various specific degenerative conditions of the C.N.S., or of the eye itself (as retinitis pigmentosa and simple glaucoma).

Acute optic neuritis

The inflammatory foci of multiple sclerosis or related (? virus) neuropathies generally cause acute optic neuritis. Very occasionally the focus is placed so near its anterior end that the engorgement may be visible ophthalmoscopically on the optic disc as a *papillitis* (this closely resembles a papilloedema due to raised intracranial pressure, but the latter is accompanied by a negligible loss of sight), otherwise it is a *retro-bulbar neuritis*, and the only visible change emerges later as a pallor of the optic disc—an 'optic atrophy', which may be very indefinite if only a few of the axon bundles have been destroyed. It is those from the central regions of the retina that are usually damaged, so that the blurred vision can be shown (by mapping the visual fields) to be due to a central or paracentral scotoma (Fig. 9.4). In the early days the eyeball may be tender, or eye movements painful due to the stretching of an inflamed optic nerve. The inflammation recedes after a week or two leaving little visual damage, but as further bouts whittle the sight away, a pallid disc may develop in later years.

CEREBRAL DISORDERS

From the lateral geniculate bodies, the visual fibres are relayed to the visual cortex through the optic radiations. Damage to these posterior fibres leads to appropriate defects in the visual fields, but without any tell-tale optic atrophy. As these fibres 'radiate' from the geniculate body, the damage is more often confined to a limited part of the fibre-bundle (whereas in the circumscribed optic tract, the whole of the appropriate half-field is usually lost). The commonest intracranial lesion to affect vision is a thrombosis of the posterior cerebral vessels, which causes a homonymous hemianopia (Fig. 9.2), with a loss of the nasal field of one eye and the corresponding temporal field of its fellow, and this may be complete, or largely restricted to the lower or upper half-fields, if only the upper or lower branches of the posterior cerebral vessels are involved. Similar field encroachments inevitably follow tumours, abscesses, fractures and other lesions of the occipital region.

Migraine is attributed to a spasm followed by vasodilatation of the cerebral arteries: when this occurs over the visual cortex, the migraine is typified by prodromal visual disturbances. The most common of these are the fortification spectra of brilliant shimmering zigzag lines, like neon signs but often of different colours; these are associated with an overall darkening of vision, or a homonymous hemianopia from which the fixation spot itself frequently escapes. After about ten minutes the vision clears, but a severe headache follows, which again may be restricted to one side or, very occasionally, may be associated with extra-ocular palsies ('ophthalmoplegic migraine'), and the patient may be incapacitated for the rest of the day. Sometimes only the prodromal visual symptoms are experienced, sometimes only the headache, and very occasionally the retinal arteries are also involved. Migraine tends to be hereditary, and also tends to start around adolescence and become less severe after middle-age.

Treatment is generally symptomatic, with rest, sedation and darkness until the attack passes or is annulled by sleep. Ergotamine tartrate or large doses of urea sometimes help, and since the attacks may be promoted by any source of nervous irritation, these should be sought, and, if found, eradicated.

FUNCTIONAL BLINDNESS

Blindness (amaurosis) or blurring of vision (amblyopia) without evident organic changes may occur in various pathological states. In uraemia *amaurosis* may be sudden and complete, but fully restored within a day or two; this is probably due to a toxic effect on the occipital cortex as in the blindness following postbasic meningitis, since in both cases the pupil reflexes are unaffected. Sudden blindness may follow severe haemorrhage (usually from uterus or intestine), one eye succeeding its fellow some days later. Sometimes a little sight returns, otherwise a dense optic atrophy develops. The term *amblyopia* is usually restricted to the congenital lowering of acuity with high unilateral refractive errors, due to suppression of an image which is grossly out of focus, and 'strabismic amblyopia' which develops in a squinting eye when the image is irreconcilably doubled. But it is also traditionally used for the impaired vision from toxic neuritis—as in 'tobacco amblyopia'.

Hysterical blindness is not uncommon, and may be perpetuated from a head injury. The blindness is usually bilateral, and when it is partial, a spiral constriction of the visual fields is classically described, the field becoming progressively smaller as it is charted round the perimeter; sometimes the eyes are rolled upwards as if in a fit, or a ptosis may be sustained to emphasize the barrier to vision. Otherwise the hysteric may signalize her escape from reality in many bizarre ways, including a squint and hallucinations (although these are more commonly found in various forms of drug addiction, organic basal lesions and the organically blind). In spite of this apparently crippling handicap, underlined by a wealth of gesture and expression, the patient manages to avoid major obstacles in her path, and the pupillary reflexes are unaffected. Indeed the psychopathic retreat from life's problems may be underwritten in a more terminal way by actually expunging the eyes, as a form of self-castration, when these are blamed as the vehicles of some spiritual or sexual lapse. The patron saint of ophthalmology, St Lucy, so expiated her sexual guilt, but God apparently gave her two replacements.

Malingering, like hysteria, may be manifested in a prolixity of ways, commonly by the false attribution of existing blemishes, or by the insertion of irritants into the conjunctival sac, but also occasionally by counterfeiting amblyopia or blindness. The diagnosis is suspected, as in hysteria, by the striking normality of the 'blind' eyes, and the antecedent circumstances (usually the desire for compensation for an alleged industrial accident); and there are various tricks by which the 'blind' eye can be demonstrated to be seeing normally.

Hallucinations (the apparent perception of an external object where none exists) and **illusions** (misinterpretations of things that are seen) may feature in many forms of functional visual disturbance. Hallucinations often fill the visual 'screen' when this has been rendered empty after some vascular occlusion, as from a giant-cell arteritis or posterior cerebral thrombosis, in which case the seen world seems to extend vaguely on into the hemianopic area. Illusions are usually toxic manifestations—the spots on the alcoholic's counterpane that turn into pink rats as delirium tremens sets in, or the macabre misinterpretations of external objects which are the reward or punishment for an overdose of L.S.D.

OCULAR NEUROSIS

In medicine at large, most symptoms are in part psycho-neurotic; and this is particularly manifest in the eye, which has always been a strongly emotive symbol of life and libido, with blindness, the traditional penalty for sexual or spiritual lapse, its recompense in myth and fable being wisdom or second-sight. So ocular neuroses abound: blurred vision, tired eyes, eye-strain, pain around or behind the eyeballs, and so on. Often these symptoms are based on real, if trifling, impediments, particularly the irritation and congestion of a mild seborrhoeic blepharitis, the nuisance of *muscae volitantes*, or the focusing effort of prolonged close work. For these symptoms spectacles are often prescribed with little organic justification, on the spurious grounds that, by 'resting' the eyes, they may 'conserve' the sight; and they may indeed be welcomed in that they provide a protective shield against the exacting world outside, particularly if the lenses are darkened to emphasize this protection.

THE SOCIAL PROBLEMS OF BLINDNESS

The world's population of blind numbers nearly twenty million; the great majority of these are in tropical and subtropical countries, where cataracts and corneal lesions abound and eye-doctors are sparse. In England there are nearly 60,000 registered as 'blind' (i.e. with vision in the better eye below 3/60), and about 20,000 on the 'partially-sighted' register (below 6/60 with full field, or up to 6/18 if gross field restriction); the large majority of these are elderly (usually with cataract, glaucoma or senile macular dystrophy). Such registration (by a consultant ophthalmologist) will ensure special schooling for those partially-sighted young, who cannot manage a normal-sighted school, and for all ages the teaching of 'Braille' (or the simplified version, 'Moon'), together with a panoply of other devices, which should ensure as far as possible full employment and contentment. And those whose sight is impaired to a lesser extent may still be supplied with 'talking books' (in cassettes) on completion of a short formal certificate.

CHAPTER 10
TROPICAL OPHTHALMOLOGY

The foregoing chapters aim to cover the field of ophthalmology as encountered in the Western world; but students in tropical and subtropical countries will need to supplement these by a basic knowledge of the eye-diseases peculiar to their own regions, and which may there provide the principal causes of loss of sight.

The eyes of such tropical and subtropical peoples have certain differences in their normal responses that should be noted. They usually become presbyopic much earlier—generally around the age of 35. Their iris, loaded with pigment cells, dilates less readily and less completely with mydriatics—a barrier to easy fundus examination and retinoscopy; and the exuberant pigment cells may spread, particularly along the penetrating scleral vessels, to give the spurious appearance of conjunctival melanosis or melanomata. This same exuberance probably explains the tendency for operative fistulae in simple glaucoma to become blocked and require repetition. On the other hand, the eyes of most coloured races are generally more resilient, and withstand a raised intra-ocular pressure with less damage to the fields of vision; and they heal more readily after injury or operation than their less pigmented fellows.

Hypovitaminosis

Undernourishment is so widespread in tropical countries, that this may justly be included as a 'tropical disease'; whilst the deficiency of vitamins A and B is the commonest cause of blindness in many such areas.

Vitamin A is a fat-soluble alcohol deriving from the vegetable pigment carotene. A-deficiency causes dessication and keratinization of skin and mucosae, which in infants particularly involves the eye, leading to rapid and permanent blindness through corneal perforation. At first the conjunctiva becomes dull, leathery and rather wrinkled, while the corneal epithelium follows suit ('xerophthalmia'), and ulceration follows. The inflammatory response is slight, so the eye may not attract attention until the iris is seen to be bulging through a wide gap in the lower central cornea.

99

If sloughing of the cornea is threatened, a large intramuscular dose (100,000 i.u.) of vitamin A may avert this disaster and save the eye; later on the vitamin can be given orally (50,000 units a day), together with dietary control (especially adequate milk).

In adults, where the skin changes are more marked than those of the cornea and conjunctiva, the other ocular manifestation—night blindness—is often the presenting feature. This can be crudely tested by noting a relative delay in discerning objects, such as the ability to count fingers, when the room is suddenly darkened.

The *vitamin B* complex is a group of water-soluble enzymes needed for intracellular metabolism; they are found in most animals and plants, and especially in cereals and yeasts. A lack of thiamine (B_1) provokes a polyneuritis, paraesthesia, weakness and loss of reflexes, including any form of ocular palsy. These signs may be submerged, in the 'wet' form of beriberi, by a presenting oedema due to heart failure.

Lack of riboflavine (B_2) presents (some weeks after any associated signs of B_1 deficiency) with angular stomatitis, glossitis, scrotal dermatitis, vascularizing keratitis, and, later, a retrobulbar neuritis; the latter may leave a permanent central or paracentral scotoma, with some corresponding optic atrophy.

Epidemic dropsy

Glaucoma is a classical feature of poisoning by argemone oil (from seeds of the Mexican poppy), which is commonly used in India and Pakistan in cooking and for anointing the body. This poison produces a gross generalized dilatation of capillaries, including those of the uvea; a glaucoma develops in consequence, with a high tension and persistent haloes, but with little conjunctival congestion and only a very gradual field loss. The glaucoma may persist, even after the poison is excluded, and it will then require control with oral acetazolamide (miotics are ineffective), or an operation if there has been a significant field loss.

Leprosy

Leprosy is found in most humid countries of the tropics and subtropics, and is usually contracted during childhood (adults having a high resistance). The eyes are involved in about a quarter of both clinical types:

The *tuberculoid(neural)* form shows scattered patches over the skin which are pale, dry and variably anaesthetic; the lids are commonly affected, with loss of lashes and eyebrows, and the skin may become so stiff and contracted that the lids cannot close, especially if the facial nerve is also damaged. Progressive corneal ulceration from exposure is thus an almost certain sequel unless the eye is protected by a tarsorrhaphy.

In the *lepromatous* form, patches also appear on the lids, but these are less well-demarcated and only an inch or two in diameter. They become increasingly prominent, forming nodules that produce ptosis rather than a lid retraction, while loss of the eyelashes and eyebrows is again a feature. In this type of leprosy the bacilli may invade the eye itself, causing episcleral nodules or a deep corneal infltrate; many cases indeed show very fine punctate corneal deposits which are symptom-free (and which lack any of the vascularization that characterizes trachoma and ariboflavinosis). The infection may spread to provoke iritis or choroiditis, or even a frank leproma may develop within the anterior chamber.

Onchocerciasis

The filaria *Onchocerca volvulus* is a frequent cause of blindness in Central Africa and Central America. The microfilariae (transmitted by the Jinja fly) spread beneath the skin and frequently (in about a third of cases) invade the cornea, causing infiltrates that resemble snowflakes; in severe infections these opacities may coalesce and obstruct the sight, or a secondary iritis may develop. The sight may also be damaged by choroido-retinal degeneration and optic atrophy (less certainly due to onchocercal infection). These ocular changes improve markedly after treatment with diethylcarbamazine (Hetrazan).

Many other tropical diseases can occasionally damage the sight, but in most cases this is too rare or coincidental to deserve emphasis here. Thus the skin of the lids commonly partakes in any generalized urticaria (as with *schistosomiasis*), and commonly suffers the bites of *insects* and *spiders*; *ticks* may adhere so firmly to the eyelid that only a hot probe or a dab of chloroform will dislodge them, just as an adherent *leech* will need a touch of salt before it releases its hold. Such bites and stings can similarly involve the conjunctiva, which may also find itself a receptacle for fly larvae (*myiasis*), or be invaded by the caterpillar hairs that provoke an *ophthalmia nodosa* (these may even penetrate the cornea to provoke nodules on the iris). The cornea may likewise be damaged by *ant* bites (mainly in infants). or by the projected venom from 'spitting' *snakes*.

Corneal ulcers also feature in *cholera*, where exposure ulceration often develops during periods of semi-coma, or in *malaria* where dendritic ulceration is a common sequel. To all these may be added a retinue of fundal changes (the retinopathy of *sickle-cell anaemia*, and so on); but, as was noted in our opening paragraph, although ophthalmology is a small speciality, the whole field of medicine lies within its frontiers.

APPENDIX 1
OPHTHALMIC QUESTIONS FROM SOME RECENT 'FINAL' EXAMINATION* PAPERS IN SURGERY

Cambridge MB, BChir

Give the causes, signs, symptoms and treatment of detachment of the retina.

A wicket-keeper is struck in the eye by a fast-rising ball. What immediate injuries may result, and how would you investigate them in hospital?

Discuss the value of the ophthalmoscope in surgical diagnosis.

Discuss . . .(a) The differential diagnosis of iridocyclitis.

Describe very briefly how you would deal with the following cases attending your surgery in private practice.

 . . . (a) Abrasions of the cornea.

Describe briefly how you would deal with the following conditions occurring in a country practice.

 . . . (a) Foreign body in the conjunctival sac.

What are the causes of a squint in an adult patient?

Enumerate the causes of a painful red eye in a young female. How is the diagnosis made?

What are the indications for corneal grafting—outline the procedure.

Describe the differential diagnosis and treatment of the watery eye.

What is the differential diagnosis between conjunctivitis and an iritis? Describe briefly how they are treated.

Write short notes on:

 . . . acute glaucoma [twice].

 . . . lacrimal duct obstruction

 . . . iridocyclitis.

 . . . squint in childhood.

 . . . the differential diagnosis between acute conjunctivitis and acute iritis (iridocyclitis].

 . . . proptosis.

---

* Acknowledgements are due to the authorities of the Universities of Cambridge, Oxford and London, and to the Committee of Management of the Examining Board in England for permission to reproduce these questions.

103

Oxford BM, BCh

Discuss the diagnosis and treatment of acute glaucoma.
What is glaucoma? How is it treated?
Write short notes on . . . Exophthalmos.

London MB, BS

Give the symptoms, signs and treatment of acute glaucoma. Describe the
causation and treatment of conjunctivitis.

Conjoint Examining Board in England for R.C.P. and R.C.S.

State how you would deal with a patient alleged to have a foreign body in
the eye.
Discuss the aetiology, diagnosis and treatment of corneal ulcer.
Discuss . . . (a) The differential diagnosis of iridocyclitis.
Describe the management and complications of injuries to the eye.
Describe the orbit and its contents, excluding the internal anatomy of the
eyeball.
Describe the causes, diagnosis and treatment of conjunctivitis.
Write short notes on:
 . . . cataract [five times].
 . . . keratitis.
 . . . acute glaucoma.
 . . . acute iridocyclitis [twice].
 . . . corneal ulcer [twice].
 . . . optic atrophy.
 . . . ectropion.
 . . . proptosis [three times].
 . . . glaucoma [five times].
 . . . ectropion.
 . . . conjunctivitis [three times].
 . . . iridocyclitis.
 . . . Meibomian cyst [twice].
 . . . Foreign-body in the eye [twice].

APPENDIX 2
MULTIPLE CHOICE QUESTIONS

Multiple Choice Questions have become a common form of test in the Final MB, and Ophthalmology is no exception. It is hoped that this Appendix will serve both to acquaint the student with the style of question he will have to face, and to further his understanding of the subject matter, as he ploughs his way through each separate chapter.

Good advice is already available by both the excellent Multiple Choice Booklets, complementary to *Lecture Notes on Clinical Medicine*, provided by Rubenstein & Wayne, and *Lecture Notes on General Surgery*, by Fleming & Stokes. Two further points concerning techniques deserve emphasis.

First, words such as 'always' and 'never' rarely apply to the discipline of medicine, and such questions should arouse strong suspicion as to their validity. In contrast, almost anything 'can' or 'may' occur. Such key words may give the answer away, even when the student does not know the content of the question.

Secondly, although blind guessing is to be discouraged, 'hunches' and 'first impressions' are more often right than wrong. Re-appraisals commonly lead to errors! It may be valuable, therefore, to assess approximately how many marks you need to ensure a pass. If you are home and dry, then taking calculated risks is unnecessary. However, if you are struggling for marks, act on 'hunches'.

Such strategy forms the basis of sound examination technique.

QUESTIONS

CHAPTER 1: answers p. 114–5

1 With respect to eye structures

1 The eye-ball is unprotected posteriorly.   F
2 Corneal ulcers usually penetrate the whole corneal thickness.   F

3 Corneal damage rarely impairs the sight. F
4 The uveal tract is continued posteriorly as the choroid. T
5 At the posterior margin of the ciliary body, the uveal tract is continued as the iris. F
6 The aqueous humour circulates from the anterior to the posterior chamber. F
7 The aqueous humour disperses from the anterior chamber via the canal of Schlemm. T
8 The ciliary muscle relaxes the suspensory ligament when it contracts. T
9 As a result of ciliary muscle contraction, the lens focuses for far-vision. F
10 Fibres from the nasal half of the retina carry impulses from the temporal half of the visual field of the same eye. T
11 The uveal tract is of ectodermal origin. F

CHAPTER 2: answers p. 115–6

1 Ptosis

1 is usually bilateral. F × T
2 may be congenital T
3 occurs as a senile myasthenia. T
4 occurring unilaterally, suggests the possibility of malignancy. T
5 is best treated by resection of some of the Levator Palpebrae of the lower tarsal plate. F

2 Styes

1 are localized infections of the glands of the lid margin. T
staph 2 external styes are usually Streptococcal in origin. F
3 external styes are best treated by incision. F
4 internal styes are infected Meibomian glands. T
5 internal styes may leave residual cysts which are characteristically painful. F

3 Blepharitis

superficial infection 1 is a localized infection of the eyelid margins. T ×
2 is often associated with Seborrhoeic Dermatitis. T
3 in its ulcerative form, involves a Staphylococcal infection. T
4 is best treated surgically. F
5 topical steroids may be of value in the Seborrhoeic type. T

4 Eyelids

1 usually evert in adults with orbicularis weakness. ⊤
2 usually evert if the tarsal conjunctival is scarred. ⊨
3 spastic entropion is best treated surgically. ⊤
4 atonic ectropion is commonly due to a flaccid orbicularis following a facial nerve palsy. ⊤ ×

Senile . more common.

5 Dacryocystitis

pneumococcus
1 in its acute form, is usually caused by the Staphylococcus. ⊤ × ⊨
2 is seen as a tender induration at the ~~lateral~~ *medial* angle of the eye. ⊤ × ⊨
3 most commonly, the chronic variety occurs in the absence of a previous acute phase. ⊨ × ⊤
4 the characteristic symptom of the chronic form is epiphora. ⊤
5 is best treated in the first instance by Dacryocysto-rhinostomy. ⊨

6 Xanthelasmata

1 occur symmetrically at the ~~lateral~~ *medial* ends of the upper or lower lids. ⊤ × ⊨
2 are commonly related to a generalized lipoidosis. ⊤ × ⊨
3 are associated with Dermato-myositis. ⊨
4 are associated with Thyrotoxicosis. ⊨

7 Exophthalmos

1 pulsating exophthalmos is characteristic of a carotico-cavernous fistula. ⊤
2 mild Dysthyroid Exophthalmos is commoner in men. ⊨
3 severe Dysthyroid Exophthalmos is commoner in women. ⊨
4 severe Dysthyroid Exophthalmos is beneficially treated by a small lateral Tarsorrhaphy. ⊤ ×⊨. *wide tars overlaps.*
5 associated lid lag in the mild form should be treated surgically. ⊨

CHAPTER 3: answers p. 116–7

1 Acute conjunctivitis

1 is usually bilateral.
2 is characterized by 'circumcorneal' injection.

3 is usually very painful.
4 is associated with only mild photophobia.
5 is usually caused by the Pneumococcus.

2 Acute Iritis

1 is usually bilateral.
2 is characterized by a dilated irregular pupil.
3 is characterized by a 'circumcorneal' injection.
4 is associated with Keratic Precipitates which cause blurring of vision.
5 is associated with posterior synechias between the iris and cornea.

3 Acute iritis

1 is most commonly caused by Exogenous infection.
2 is associated classically with Crohn's disease.
3 may be complicated by both Glaucoma and Cataract.
4 should be treated with topical cortico-steroids.
5 should *not* be treated with atropine, as acute Glaucoma may be precipitated.

4 Acute glaucoma is characterized by

1 mild pain, characteristically relieved by aspirin.
2 minimal loss of vision.
3 a fixed semi-dilated pupil which will not respond to light.
4 a shallow anterior chamber.
5 stony hard ocular tension.

5 Closed-angle glaucoma

1 occurs especially in myopic patients.
2 is characterized by bouts of raised tension.
3 is precipitated by pupillary dilation.
4 occurs in eyes with a shallow anterior chamber.
5 tends to occur most commonly in the very old patient.

6 In the treatment of acute glaucoma

1 Acetazolamide helps to constrict the pupil.

2 Glycerol may be of value in dehydrating the eye.
3 Pilocarpine drops should be inserted as soon as possible.
4 Peripheral Iridectomy should be performed as soon as possible.
5 Pilocarpine drops should be continued after the initial attack.

7 Acute keratitis

1 usually presents as a corneal ulcer.
2 is more commonly endogenous in origin.
3 in its endogenous form, starts in the superficial layers of the cornea.

8 With respect to corneal ulcers.

1 the marginal type are usually caused by a Staphylococcal conjunctival infection.
2 marginal ulcers are usually multiple.
3 marginal ulcers characteristically cause ultimate impairment of vision.
4 central ulcers are usually single.
5 central ulcers are most commonly caused by pneumococcal infection.
6 central ulcers are associated with facial palsy.

9 In the treatment of corneal ulcers

1 the drugs used are essentially the same as for combined conjunctivitis and iritis.
2 Idoxuridene is specifically of value for dendritic ulcers.
3 steroid drops are contra-indicated for dendritic ulcers.
4 Carbolization is of value if the ulcer is indolent.
5 Tarsorrhaphy many be required if corneal sensation is lowered.

CHAPTER 4: answers p. 118–9

1 Cataracts

1 are the commonest cause of certifiable blindness in the UK.
2 classically present with gradual failure of vision.
3 are seen as a white opacity within the pupil.
4 are seen ophthalmoscopically as a silhouette against the red fundus reflex.
5 are best treated by steroid drops.

2 Cataracts are associated with

1 Neonatal hypo-calcaemia.
2 Rubella.
3 Hypo-thyroidism.
4 Juvenile and Maturity-onset Diabetes.
5 Galactosaemia.
6 Chloroquine therapy.
7 Chloramphenicol eye drops.
8 Dystrophia Myotonica.

3 In simple Glaucoma

1 the anterior chamber is narrowed.
2 there is probably a senile sclerotic change in the smaller intra-ocular vessels.
3 the disc is cupped, white and atrophic.
4 the eyeball is stony hard.
5 visual loss starts as a scotoma.

4 The treatment of Simple Glaucoma

1 is essentially the same as for acute episodes of closed-angle glaucoma.
2 usually involves sclerectomy.
3 may be helped by neutral adrenalin drops.
4 is curative.

5 Macular degeneration (dystrophy)

1 causes a unilateral central Scotoma.
2 can occur in infancy.
3 is associated with Tay-Sachs disease.
4 may be mimicked by Chloroquine therapy.
5 calls for telescopic spectacles in most cases.

6 Retinitis pigmentosa

1 causes a loss of central vision.
2 is a cause of night-blindness.
3 affects the posterior pole of the fundus.

4 commences in adolescence.
5 causes progressive optic atrophy.
6 is a genetically determined disease.

CHAPTER 5: answers p. 119

1 Sudden loss of sight may occur with

1 Glaucoma.
2 Central retinal artery thrombosis.
3 Vitreous haemorrhage.
4 Temporal arteritis.

2 The following are characteristic of a diabetic retinopathy

1 Micro-aneurysms.
2 Dot and blot haemorrhages.
3 Arterio-venous nipping.
4 Cotton wool exudates.
5 Papilloedema.

3 Central retinal vein thrombosis.

1 is commonest in the elderly.
2 is characterized by a cherry-red spot at the macula.
3 is characterized by subsequent new vessel formation at the disc.
4 is associated with simple Glaucoma.
5 responds well to obliteration of the vessels by a laser or photo-coagulator beam.
6 usually involves the macula, when the upper temporal vein is affected.

4 Retinal detachments

1 may be initiated by minimal trauma.
2 are commonly bilateral.
3 are signalled by a characteristic prodromal visual disturbance.
4 are seen as a bulging opalescent sheet ballooning into the vitreous.
5 should be managed conservatively.

5 Regarding malignant tumours of the eye

1 Retinoblastoma may present as glaucoma.
2 Malignant melanoma is relatively slow growing.
3 Retinoblastoma presents in the elderly.
4 Malignant melanoma presents in infancy.
5 Retinoblastoma in the first eye is usually be treated by radio-therapy.
6 Retinoblastoma characteristically metastasizes to the liver.
7 Retinoblastoma has a familial association.

CHAPTER 6: answers p. 120

1 Regarding contusion of the eye

1 eyelid haematomas should be evacuated.
2 sub-conjunctival haemorrhages are usually spontaneous.
3 sub-conjunctival haemorrhages usually involve the whole eye.
4 sub-conjunctival haemorrhages are symptomless.
5 traumatic hyphaemas should be treated by bed rest.
6 lens dislocations are usually complete.
7 retinal haemorrhages usually impair vision.
8 optic nerve compression usually results in early blindness.

2 Blow-out orbital fractures

1 are nearly always associated with sub-conjunctival haemorrhage.
2 are recognized easily on X-ray.
3 heal without surgery.
4 are often accompanied by diplopia.
5 may result in a loss of sensation over the distribution of the intra-orbital nerve.

CHAPTER 7: answers p. 120

1 With regard to refractive errors

1 Presbyopia is an inadequacy of accommodation.
2 Presbyopia is corrected by concave reading spectacles.
3 Hypermetropia is corrected by convex spectacle lenses.
4 In myopia, the eyeball is too short.

5 The optic disc in myopia simulates papilloedema.
6 In Astigmatism, the eyeball is flattened.

CHAPTER 8: answers p. 120–1

1 The following are true of concomitant squint

1 usually develops during the first few years of life.
2 diplopia is absent.
3 both eyes have full movement if tested separately.
4 the eyes generally adopt a position of relative divergence.
5 is best treated by occlusion of the worse eye.

2 The following are true of paralytic squint

1 diplopia is maximum when looking in the direction of action of the paralysed muscle.
2 the image furthest from the midline arises from the unaffected eye.
3 the false image is always peripheral.
4 the diplopia is usually of gradual onset.
5 the diplopia disappears on covering either eye.

3 The following are true of nystagmus

1 Ocular nystagmus is usually vertical.
2 Ocular nystagmus is characteristically irregular.
3 the direction is named after the slow phase.
4 it is more pronounced when the patient looks in the direction of the slow phase.
5 Nystagmoid jerks are usually pathological.

4 Horner's syndrome is characterized by

1 Ptosis.
2 Miosis
3 Exophthalmos
4 Anhidrosis.
5 Contra-lateral pupillary dilation.

CHAPTER 9: answers p. 121–2

1 The following are causes of Papilloedema

1 Retinal venous obstruction.
2 Anaemia.
3 Severe diabetes.
4 Raised intra-cranial pressure.
5 Arterial hypertension.
6 Hypercapnia.
7 Retrobulbar neuritis.

2 The following are causes of optic atrophy

1 Papilloedema.
2 Multiple sclerosis.
3 Pituitary tumour.
4 Diabetes.
5 Retinal artery thrombosis.
6 Choroido-retinitis.
7 Hypermetropia.
8 Paget's disease.
9 Anaemia.
10 Glaucoma.
11 Lead poisoning.
12 Tobacco smoking.
13 Optic radiation damage.

3 Regarding patterns of visual field loss

1 Tunnel vision may be caused by glaucoma.
2 Central scotoma results from retrobulbar retinitis.
3 Bitemporal hemianopias are caused by pituitary tumours.
4 Homonymous hemianopias result from temporal lobe tumours.
5 Tract lesions posterior to the chiasma cause a quadrantic hemianopia.

ANSWERS
CHAPTER 1

1   1 FALSE. It is unprotected *anteriorly* where the convex corneal window lies.

2 FALSE. This is rare.

3 FALSE. This is relatively common, especially if the resultant opaque scars are centrally placed.

4 TRUE.

5 FALSE. It is from the *anterior* margin.

6 FALSE. From the posterior to the anterior chamber.

7 TRUE.

8 TRUE.

9 FALSE. The lens focuses for Near-Vision.

10 TRUE.

11 FALSE. It is a mesodermal sheet.

CHAPTER 2

1 1 TRUE.

2 TRUE.

3 TRUE.

4 TRUE.

5 FALSE. It is the upper plate which should be resected.

2 1 TRUE.

2 FALSE. Staphylococcal.

3 FALSE. No treatment is necessary. They usually discharge themselves. Heat and antibiotic ointment may be of value.

4 TRUE.

5 FALSE. They are usually symptomless.

3 1 FALSE. It is a generalized infection.

2 TRUE.

3 TRUE.

4 FALSE. Frequent shampoos, alkaline lotions and drops or ointments containing cortico-steroid and antibiotics are all of value.

5 TRUE. They should, however, be used with caution as there is a risk of precipitating Simple Glaucoma.

4 1 TRUE.

2 FALSE. Inverts.

3 TRUE.

4 FALSE. A senile loss of tone of the lower lid muscles is more common.

5 1 FALSE. Pneumococcus.

 2 FALSE. It occurs at the medial angle.

 3 TRUE.

 4 TRUE.

 5 FALSE. Syringing should be initially tried.

6 1 FALSE. They occur at the medial ends.

 2 FALSE. This is rare.

 3 FALSE.

 4 FALSE.

7 1 TRUE.

 2 FALSE. Women.

 3 FALSE. Affects sexes equally.

 4 FALSE. This is beneficial for the mild variety. Wide Tarsorrhaphy and even orbital decompression may be required for the severe type.

 5 FALSE. Guanethidine drops should be tried.

CHAPTER 3

1 1 TRUE.

 2 FALSE. This is characteristic of acute iritis and acute glaucoma.

 3 FALSE. More a sensation of grittiness than true pain.

 4 TRUE.

 5 FALSE. This only accounts for the rare severe bouts. *Staph. Aureus* is the usual pathogen.

2 1 FALSE.

 2 FALSE. The pupil is constricted.

 3 TRUE.

 4 TRUE.

 5 FALSE. These are the rarer *anterior* synechias. Posterior synechias are adhesions between the iris and the anterior lens surface.

3 1 FALSE. The cause is usually obscure.

 2 FALSE. It rarely occurs in Crohn's disease.

 3 TRUE.

 4 TRUE.

 5 FALSE. Atropine-induced glaucoma is very rare and only occurs in patients with very shallow anterior chambers.

4 1 FALSE. The pain is most severe, enough to make the patient vomit.

2 FALSE. Vision may be reduced to a bare perception of light.

3 TRUE.

4 TRUE.

5 TRUE.

5 1 FALSE. It is commoner in hypermetropes, whose smaller eyeballs have shallower anterior chambers.

2 TRUE.

3 TRUE.

4 TRUE.

5 FALSE. It is commoner in the middle-aged.

6 1 FALSE. Acetazolamide is a carbonic anhydrase inhibitor and consequently cuts down the secretion from the ciliary body.

2 TRUE.

3 TRUE.

4 FALSE. Only after medical treatment has controlled the attack.

5 TRUE. This is necessary to maintain a constricted pupil (unless and until peripheral iridotomy is done).

7 1 TRUE.

2 FALSE. Exogenous causes are much commoner since the cornea is exposed to trauma and infection.

3 FALSE. It starts in the deep layers.

8 1 TRUE.

2 TRUE.

3 FALSE.

4 TRUE.

5 FALSE. Herpes Simplex Virus is a commoner cause.

6 TRUE. The lids cannot adequately protect the cornea.

9 1 TRUE.

2 TRUE.

3 TRUE. They may promote an extension of the ulcer.

4 TRUE.

5 TRUE.

CHAPTER 4

1 1 FALSE. Senile macular degeneration is commoner.
2 TRUE.
3 TRUE.
4 TRUE.
5 FALSE. The only treatment is to remove them surgically.

2 1 TRUE.
2 TRUE.
3 FALSE.
4 TRUE.
5 TRUE.
6 FALSE.
7 FALSE.
8 TRUE.

3 1 FALSE. It is of normal depth.
2 TRUE.
3 TRUE.
4 FALSE. Although moderately hard, it is not so tense and stony as in an acute attack of glaucoma.
5 TRUE.

4 1 TRUE.
2 FALSE. This is a last resort.
3 TRUE.
4 FALSE. The degenerative process often slowly progresses, eventually destroying the sight.

5 1 FALSE. It is usually bilateral.
2 TRUE.
3 TRUE.
4 TRUE.
5 FALSE. A simple hand-magnifying lens often serves these elderly patients best.

6 1 FALSE. The loss is peripheral.
2 TRUE.

3 FALSE. The black pigment is deposited over the whole fundus *except* the posterior pole.

4 TRUE.

5 TRUE.

6 TRUE.

CHAPTER 5

1 1 FALSE.

   2 TRUE.

   3 TRUE.

   4 TRUE.

2 1 TRUE.

   2 TRUE.

   3 FALSE. This is characteristic of hypertension.

   4 TRUE.

   5 FALSE. This occurs in Grade 4 hypertension.

3 1 TRUE.

   2 FALSE. This is characteristic of central retinal artery thrombosis.

   3 TRUE.

   4 TRUE.

   5 FALSE. Treatment is of no avail.

   6 TRUE.

4 1 TRUE.

   2 TRUE.

   3 TRUE. Sudden flashes and floating opacities before the eye.

   4 TRUE.

   5 FALSE. Without surgery, the detachment normally becomes complete, and the eye blind.

5 1 TRUE.

   2 FALSE.

   3 FALSE. Early infancy is the rule.

   4 FALSE. Middle-age is the rule.

   5 FALSE. Enucleation is usually required.

   6 FALSE. It travels up the optic nerve to the brain.

   7 TRUE.

CHAPTER 6

1 1 FALSE. NO TREATMENT IS NECESSARY.

2 TRUE.

3 FALSE.

4 TRUE.

5 TRUE.

6 FALSE. They are usually partial.

7 FALSE. This is rare. Vision is impaired only if the haemorrhages overlie the macula.

8 TRUE.

2 1 TRUE. A rare case of a valid 'always'.

2 TRUE.

3 TRUE. But may trap the Inferior Rectus muscle.

4 TRUE.

5 TRUE.

CHAPTER 7

1 1 TRUE.

2 FALSE. Convex.

3 TRUE.

4 FALSE. It is too long.

5 FALSE. This is the case in Hypermetropia.

6 TRUE.

CHAPTER 8

1 1 TRUE.

2 TRUE.

3 TRUE.

4 FALSE. Convergence.

5 FALSE. The better eye is occluded, thereby forcing the child to use the squinting eye.

2 1 TRUE.

2 FALSE. It arises from the paralysed eye.

3 TRUE. Another rare case of a valid 'always'.

4 FALSE. It is usually of sudden onset.

5 TRUE.

3 1 FALSE. Usually horizontal.

2 FALSE. Regular pendulum-like movements.

3 FALSE. Fast phase.

4 FALSE. Fast phase.

5 FALSE. They are commonly produced in the normal eyes.

4 1 TRUE.

2 TRUE.

3 FALSE. Enophthalmos.

4 TRUE.

5 FALSE.

CHAPTER 9

1 1 TRUE.

2 TRUE.

3 FALSE.

4 TRUE.

5 TRUE.

6 TRUE.

7 TRUE.

2 1 TRUE. In this secondary optic atrophy, the disc edge is blurred.

2 TRUE. Primary optic atrophy; disc margin sharp.

3 TRUE. Arises from pressure on the optic nerve.

4 TRUE.

5 TRUE. ⎱
6 TRUE. ⎰ A 'consecutive' optic atrophy.

7 FALSE.

8 TRUE. By compression.

9 TRUE. ⎱
10 TRUE. ⎰ Ischaemic atrophy.

11 TRUE. Toxic atrophy.
12 TRUE.

13 FALSE.

3 1 TRUE.

2 TRUE.

3 TRUE.

4 FALSE. These produce quadrantic hemianopias.

5 FALSE. These produce homonymous hemianopias.

APPENDIX 3
SHORT GLOSSARY

AMAUROSIS Blindness, without evident organic cause

AMBLYOPIA Impaired vision without evident organic cause

APHAKIA The absence of the lens (from its place within the eye)

BUPHTHALMOS Congenital glaucoma

CHALAZION Meibomian cyst (cyst within the tarsal plate)

COLOBOMA Gap in the uveal 'cup', usually as sector-shaped defect of iris or choroid

COMMOTIO Pigmentary disturbance of retina after blunt trauma

DACRYOCYSTITIS Inflammation of the tear sac

ECTROPION Eversion of eyelid

ENTROPION Inversion of eyelid

EPIPHORA Watering eye (overflow of tears)

EVISCERATION Removal of eyeball contents from within the sclera

GLAUCOMA Damage to sight associated with raised intra-ocular pressure

HORDEOLUM External stye (furuncle at root of eyelash)

HYPHAEMA Blood in anterior chamber

HYPOPYON Pus in anterior chamber

IRIDENCLEISIS Operation for simple glaucoma, inserting 'wick' of iris tissue in a limbal incision

IRIDODIALYSIS Tear along iris root from trauma

IRIDODONESIS Tremulous iris, through lack of posterior support from lens

MUSCAE VOLITANTES Wispy opacities which float before vision in healthy eyes

PHTHISIS BULBI Shrinkage of eyeball (following endophthalmitis)

PINGUECULA Fatty thickening of bulbar conjunctiva to either side of cornea

PROPTOSIS Forward protrusion of eyeball

PTERYGIUM Opaque thickening at limbus which spreads from either side into cornea

SCOTOMA Patch of impaired vision in visual field

STRABISMUS Squint; deviation of the (normally parallel) visual axes

STREPTOTHRIX Fungus with branching threads, which causes 'actino-mycosis'; concretions may block lacrimal canaliculi

SYMBLEPHARON Adherence of eyelid onto eyeball

INDEX